Pandemic Effects
Mental Health in Young Children

Araceli Hansen

Preface

When people talk about covid-19, what are they talking about? The rising numbers of cases and deaths? The beloved ones lost to the pandemic? Secondary disasters caused by the pandemic? The discrimination and racism that can be worse than the virus? Vaccines and possible side effects of vaccines?

Although the pandemic is about to approach its third year, and in most parts of the world the impact of the pandemic on daily life seems to be receding and people are regaining a sense of what life was like before the pandemic, everyone knows something is different. Do you still remember your state of mind at the beginning of the pandemic, under all the uncertainty? Have you ever thought about how Covid-19 has made a difference in your life? My project is a podcast based on an oral history of that uncertainty and change.

Table of Content

Introduction of the project 5

Narrators' Introduction 8

Podcast Info 11

Transcription and translation 12

    Vol-1 Evan 13

    Vol-2 Keke 27

    Vol-3 71 50

    Vol-4 Zoey 78

    Vol-5 Lily 97

Reflective essay 110

    Dealing with different interviewees 110

    Relationship with my narrators 115

    Self-censorship in China 118

    Oral history and podcast 120

Works Cited 124

Introduction of the project

Since the pandemic, I have increasingly found that in the Chinese context, people are often reminded to see the deeper suffering of more vulnerable groups. College students who are locked in their dorm rooms are asked not to complain, but to see the elderly who are starving during the lockdown. People even comforted those who are suffering pay cuts because of the pandemic with the fact that there are more people out of work with absolutely no income. Given this background, the students who are studying abroad or planning to study abroad are considered to be a group with more financial security and family support so that they can enjoy more social capital to overcome uncertainty. And thus, their narratives of pandemic disruption are often criticized as making too much fuss.

However, even without deep suffering, collective emotions and individualized difficulties did exist among this group. Their voices should also be part of the historical narrative. As a member of this group, I would like to record some of the voices belonging to them. I believe this can be meaningful as some kind of group memory.

According to the UNESCO Institute for Statistics, China has over 1 million mobile students abroad. (*Global Flow of Tertiary-Level Students*) Although this accounts for a very small portion of China's huge population, it is still a large group of people. Students with different educational backgrounds and life experiences will naturally have very different stories and ideas. I was unable to cover every type of person in my interviews, so I chose as my interviewees the people with the most similar backgrounds to mine: those who got their bachelor's degrees from a Chinese university in summer 2020 and initially planned to enroll in a foreign university for further study.

Almost three years ago when the pandemic suddenly hit, we were at some kind of crossroads in our lives. We all got offers from our dream graduate schools. Because of the pandemic, some of us had a gap year that we had never planned for and enrolled in 2021. Some of us, facing similar circumstances, made very different choices. Many of us took a completely different path in life than we expected because of these choices. All these essential decisions were made under great uncertainty and with our forecasts of the future world at the time. I did oral history interviews with these students, helping them look back at the decisions they made. I listened to their stories and recorded the changes in their lives and thoughts over the past years. I then worked with them to produce a podcast with these interviews to share some of their stories and insights--if recording and archiving oral histories is about self-documentation and reflection for them, then the podcast format may lead to more resonation between audience and narrators.

In addition, I find my project could be helpful for younger students, especially those who are in their senior or junior year. They are also at a crossroads in their lives, facing a similar situation as us in 2020. Recently, some of them consulted me about studying abroad during the pandemic, and I also saw some of them asking for suggestions on social media and online international student forums. I could not really give any suggestions but only share my experiences and thoughts. However, my experience alone is quite partial, and I can only help very few people. In this way, I hope to share some more different experiences and perspectives with this group through this podcast, which may be helpful for them to make a more well-informed decision.

Narrators' Introduction

I conducted 8 interviews in the past 10 months on their life since 2020. After discussing with my interviewees, I chose five of the interviews to edit into podcasts, with each episode lasting 10-25 minutes.

Since all of my interviewees are ordinary people, although they are willing to share their experiences and insights, they don't want to be famous for participating in this podcast (This may stem from overly optimistic estimates of subscriptions to this podcast though) or to be cyber abused for having some of their statements misunderstood. We decided to use nicknames for them in the podcast and hide some personal information. And before releasing each episode, I double-checked with them. Below are the basic introductions of the five interviewees (all the information I provide here has their permission):

Evan: A master's student at the University of Sydney. He graduated from Huazhong University of Science and Technology with a bachelor's degree in computer science. Due to the travel restriction, Evan applied for a deferral and found a job in a state-owned company as a software engineer. He quit his job after one year of working, but instead of leaving for Australia immediately, he took online classes at home to wait for a better opportunity for international travel.

Keke: A master's student majoring in Public Policy at the University of Pennsylvania. She also holds a dual degree in History and International Politics from Peking University.

Facing the pandemic, Keke decided to stay in China and take online classes and do some internships at the same time, and eventually completed her post-grad education fully online. As a Wuhaner, she also witnessed the entire process of the pandemic getting worse till the city was locked down for several months and shared those memories with me.

71[1]: A master's student in the East Asian Languages and Cultures Program at Columbia University. Before entering Columbia University, she majored in Biological Science and Chinese Literature at Peking University. 71 had a gap year because she didn't want to take online classes. Right before the winter break in 2021, she unexpectedly tested positive for Covid-19, which she didn't dare to tell her family.

Zoey: Zoey graduated from a college in Shanghai as an undergraduate and the University of Michigan, Ann Arbor as a graduate student. After a year of online, she finally came to the United States and took the second half of classes of her master's program onsite. In her first year of the master's program, she often needed to stay up very late at night to take classes due to the time difference. For this reason, she even moved to live in the countryside for some days. At the time of this interview, Zoey had graduated and returned to Shanghai to work.

---

[1] She got this nickname because the pronunciation of her Chinese name is very similar to 71 in Chinese.

Lily: Lily graduated from Nanjing University in 2020. She initially planned to go to Hong Kong or Singapore for a master's degree and did receive some offers. However, the uncertainty of the pandemic made her reject all the offers and go back to her hometown. She is now working as a civil servant in the local government. She has given up the idea of studying abroad but is thinking about attending a part-time master's program in China.

Podcast Info

I've uploaded all five episodes of the podcast. The podcasts are updated simultaneously on the Apple podcast and two Chinese podcast platforms, Xiao Yuzhou 小宇宙 (Little Universe) and Himalaya based on the audience and other considerations.

The link to the Apple podcast channel is https://podcasts.apple.com/us/podcast/the-two-years-stolen/id1651221728, and the access to the other two platforms is as below.

Scan the QR code to listen to the Podcast

Transcription and translation

Since all of my interviewees are non-English native speakers, they may not express themselves in English as well as they do in Chinese. I tried to avoid the influence of language by letting them choose the language they prefer. Plus, considering most of my target audiences for the podcast may also be Chinese, I finally decided to conduct all the interviews in Chinese. For the non-Chinese speaking audience that may exist, I transcribed and translated the contents of the podcasts and attached the document to each episode.

Translating was a painful process. Sometimes my interviewees would use some Chinese common sayings or internet slang, which increased the difficulty of translating. Sometimes there are expressions that can only be perceived but cannot be described with words. Any translation would cut down or even distort the real meaning the interviewees would like to deliver.

Other times the interviews will involve companies and people that only Chinese people know about. I need to figure out which content may not be understood by non-native Chinese audiences and add footnotes for them. Although I had received a primary qualification in China regarding Chinese and English translation, I can hardly say that my translation of these interviews was entirely satisfying. But I still hope to at least help the non-Chinese speakers to basically understand the conversation between me and the interviewees.

Below are the transcription and translation of the five episodes.

Vol-1 Evan

何凯前往澳大利亚的 Evan，最后线下上了多久的课程？

What made Evan, who was waiting for an opportunity to go to Australia, end up taking classes fully online?

Evan: A master's student at the University of Sydney. He graduated from Huazhong University of Science and Technology with a bachelor's degree in computer science. Due to the travel restriction, Evan applied for a deferral and found a job in a state-owned company as a software engineer. He quit his job after one year of working, but instead of leaving for Australia immediately, he took online classes at home to wait for a better opportunity for international travel.

[00:00:00.00] (Music)

[00:00:04.26] VoiceOver: 欢迎来到 The Two Year Stolen，我是 Yiwen。

Welcome to The Two Year Stolen, I'm Yiwen.

[00:00:15.27] VoiceOver: 这一期的受访者是我的发小，我二十多年的好朋友 Evan。Evan 本科毕业于华中科技大学，现在是悉尼大学的一名学生。

The interviewee of this episode is my childhood friend Evan, whom I have known for more than 20 years. Evan graduated from Huazhong University of Science and Technology as an undergraduate. He is now a graduate student at The University of Sydney.

[00:00:26.05] (Music)

[00:00:29.20] VoiceOver: 谈及出留学，Evan 表示自己很早就已经萌生了出国留学的想法，但真正付诸实践，要等到大四上学期。

When talking about studying abroad, Evan said he had the idea of studying abroad very early, but he didn't really put it into practice until the first semester of his senior year.

[00:00:38.22] Evan: 大概是在大二的时候，曾经听到一个留学的学长回来做讲座。当时觉得他很潇洒。

When I was in my sophomore year, I heard an alumnus who had studied abroad come back to give a lecture. At that time, I thought he was so cool.

[00:00:45.29] Yiwen: 这个潇洒是指哪方面？

In what aspect did you think he was cool?

[00:00:47.17] Evan: 这个对于所有工程师来说其实都一样，觉得他的这个思想，或者说，他提出的一些点，提出的一些这个知识。当时听他做的关于这个 JavaScript 的一个讲座，觉得挺精彩的，这个和国内的研究生学长他们普遍反映的那种情况不太一样，所以我就希望能够到国外去见识见识。但是，真正付诸实施还是在，emmm，大四的时候。

This is actually the same for all engineers. I think his ideas, or some of the points he raised, and some of his knowledge (were cool). At that time, he gave us a lecture about JavaScript, and it was wonderful. It was so different from what the domestic graduate students generally talked about. So, I hoped to be able to go abroad to widen my knowledge. However, the time I really put this idea into practice was in the, emmm, senior year.

[00:01:17.21] VoiceOver: 在决定出国留学之前，Evan 还曾考虑过直接就业或是在国内考研。

Before he decided to study abroad, Evan had also considered finding a job directly after graduation or entering a graduate school in China.

[00:01:23.09] Evan: 其实关于考研的话题，在这个，大二的时候，呃，就已经有过这样的想法。但是最终还是没有付诸实施。主要是因为，这个，在九、十月份的时候，emmm，再去准备这个已经，嗯，已经来不及了。emmm，当时在这个是工作还是继续读研的这个问题上，嗯，纠缠了一段时间。我在那会儿的认识就是，因为从这个，业界来看，很多这个大专的人，都可以去写代码，对所以我当时认为，而且网上也有很多言（论）、观点认为就是，计算机专业是不是有必要读研究生，研究生能够给你带来什么？我当时受到其中一些观点的影响，认为这个研究生不是很必要。但是就是在这个纠结的过程中，其实它需要很多时间，你一会儿要准备这个，一会儿要准备这个，所以本质上，秋招和这个考研是都错过了。当然这是一点很后悔的情况。现在就不谈了。而且为什么选择出国而不是接着考研，其中也有一个原因就是从时间上讲，我出国一年半，和国内读三年，因为我还gap了一年，甚至还比他们早半年毕业。时间上讲是差不多的，我会和他们同时面对这个秋招和春招。所以当时就这个，萌生了，呃，这个，出国留学的想法。

In fact, on the topic of entering a graduate school in China, it was, in the sophomore year, uh, I already had such an idea. But in the end, I didn't put it into practice. The main reason is that, is that, it was in September and October, emmm, and it was too late to prepare for the Graduate school Entrance Exam. Emm, I was, at that time, I hesitated between pursuing a higher degree and going to work, I hesitated for some time. My understanding at that time was that, from the industry's point of view, many junior college graduates also know coding. There are also many words and opinions on the Internet that it's not necessary for CS majors to enter graduate school, and the graduate school can bring you so little promotion. At that time, I was influenced by some of these views, and I thought that this graduate school was not very necessary. The torn process is a waste of time that you have to prepare for one thing for a while, and another thing for another while. Essentially, I missed both the fall recruitment and the graduate school entrance exam. It's quite regrettable, and I don't want to talk too much. And another reason why I chose to study abroad was the time issue. If I study abroad for one and a half years, plus one year of gap year, I can even graduate half a year earlier than my classmates who enter domestic graduate school for three years. We would graduate almost the same time and face the same fall and spring recruitment. So then, under this situation, uh, I finally decided to study abroad.

[00:02:51.22] VoiceOver: 而由于提交申请时疫情已经爆发，在考虑去哪个国家时，Evan 的选择很大程度上受到了疫情因素的影响。

And since the pandemic has already happened when Evan submitted his applications, his choice was heavily influenced by the pandemic when considering which country to go to.

[00:03:00.00] Evan: 当时的情况是这样的，就是在一、二月份的时候，我先交了英联邦国家的这个申请，然后在准备的同时，我同时也在想就是最好是能够是去美国。因为计算机领域最先进的地方还，肯定还是美国，对。但是问题就是在 20 年初的时候疫情比较严重，当时是我们的国家比较，比较严重，emmm，但是总体来说这个问题不大，因为我可以在家里这个，准备这个出国留学的事宜。但是随着时

间推移，大概到了三、四月份的时候美国的疫情就比较严重起来了。就是一方面这个准备材料也需要跑这儿跑那儿的，但是当时他也封锁了，同时看到美国的疫情就觉得这个申请可能不是很有意义了，未来的一两年可能都去不了，那这个时候，嗯，其实我已经拿到了这个澳大利亚那里的 offer，然后如果想要再去美国的话，就不知道会这个要把这个留学计划推迟到猴年马月，所以就暂时这个搁置了这个去美国的计划。

The situation at that time was like, that was, in January and February, I first submitted the applications for the Commonwealth countries. And while I was preparing the application materials, I was also thinking that it would be better to go to the United States. But the problem was that the pandemic was more serious in our country at the beginning of 2020, emmm but in general, this was not a big deal, because I could stay at home and prepare for the applications. But as time went on, around March and April, the pandemic in the United States became more serious. On the one hand, I had to run here and there to prepare the documents, but at that time, it was locked down everywhere. On the other hand, considering the situation in the United States, I thought that this application might not be very meaningful, because I might not be able to go in the next one or two years. And at this time, well, actually I had already gotten the offer from Australia, and if I still chose to go to the United States instead, I didn't know that I would have to postpone this study abroad plan. So, I temporarily shelved this plan of going to the United States.

[00:04:09.06] VoiceOver: 疫情也让 Evan 做出了先去工作一段时间的决定。

The pandemic also made Evan make the decision to first work for some time.

[00:04:14.00] Yiwen: 悉尼大学的学制是⋯

The length of schooling at the University of Sydney is…

[00:04:17.00] Evan: 一般是，呃，一年半到两年。也就是说我必须要匀出一段比较完整的，比较长的时间出来。所以这就让我想，当时的想法是在 21，21 年年底之前也不一定疫情能够得到缓解。所以我的想法就是先 gap 一年，找一份工作，做一下，然后再利用后面的时间出去留学。

It's usually, uh, a year and a half to two years. That means I had to leave a more continuous, and kind of long period of time out for school. So, I was thinking, my idea at that time was that the pandemic may not be alleviated until 2021, the end of 2021. So, my idea was to gap for a year, get a job, work for some time, and then go abroad for higher education.

[00:04:38.04] Yiwen: 找工作大概是在什么时候开始，去投简历？

When did you begin to search for a job, like sending out resumes?

[00:04:40.29] Evan: 当时其实春招也过得差不多了，在互联网企业的春招。这个就要到后来了。因为我先去一家本地的企业实习了一段时间，大概到了 5 月份、6 月份。这个时候，其实当时忙着交毕业论文，然后做那个答辩。直到这个，六月，六月初，这时候才想着去，真正找一份工作干一下。结果问题就是，那会儿其实已经错过春招了。所以就，还剩下一些国企，或者是其他单位可能会招 IT 行业的从业的人员。所以我就去，留意了一下。然后在这个 7 月中旬是正式入职。

At that time, in fact, the spring recruitment is almost over, I mean the spring recruitment of IT companies. It was the later story. Because I first interned at a local company for a period of time, till May or June. Then I was busy with my bachelor's thesis and the oral defense. It was not until June, early June, that I thought about really looking for a job to do. The result was that the problem was, at that time I have actually missed the spring recruitment. But there were still some state-owned companies left, or government departments might need some IT employees. So, I paid attention to these places. Then it was in the middle of July, I was officially on board.

[00:05:23.20] Yiwen: 所以，其实你在 20 年年初做申请的时候，你其实也没有考虑过要先找工作？

So, when you were applying for graduate programs at the beginning of 2020, you didn't think about finding a job?

[00:05:30.15] Evan: 对，当时的想法就是，希望一毕业就能够衔接上去上课，但是由于疫情的问题，只好在毕业之后先找一份工作干一干。

Yes. My idea at that time was I hoped I could enter the graduate right after my graduation from undergraduate. However, due to the pandemic, I had to find a job after graduation.

[00:05:39.16] Yiwen: 你是先找到工作然后再决定 gap，还是决定了 gap 之后再去找工作？

Did you find a job first and then decide to have a gap year or the opposite?

[00:05:44.21] Evan: 说起来也不是那么巧。就是找到工作之后，怎么说呢，也不是说是当时奔着 gap 去找工作，或者冲着工作去找 gap。只是找到工作之后忽然发现，"哦！原来我还可以 gap 一年！"所以我就直接，就直接去工作了。

It was not that coincidental. It was just that after finding a job, how to say, it was not that I was looking for a job with the intention of a gap year or looking for a gap year with the intention of a job, it was just that after finding a job, I suddenly realized, "Oh! I can gap for a year!" So, I just went straight to work.

[00:06:02.28] Yiwen: 所以你去找工作的时候，你是抱着我可能要放弃这个 offer 明年重新申请的这种想法？

So, when you were searching for a job, you were holding the idea of giving up this school offer and applying again the next year?

[00:06:08.03] Evan: 是的是的。还有一个想法。就是为什么说后来只工作了一年就这个离开了呢？其实当时的想法就是，发现这个学历的重要性，尤其是在这种国有的企业，他们对学历的看重和这个私企对学历的看重不太一样。私企里面可能说，只要你有本事，只要你掌握了一定的专业技能，那么你就可以这个爬得很顺利。但是在国企里面，职称之类的东西是和这个学历是密切挂钩的。

Yes, yes. And I have another idea. Why did I leave after working for only one year? In fact, at that time, I found the importance of this degree, especially in the state-owned enterprises, they attach much more importance to the degree than the private companies. In private companies, they may say, as long as you have the ability, as long as you have honed certain professional skills, then you can get promotions very smoothly. But in state-owned enterprises, titles and other things are closely linked to the educational background.

[00:06:37.08] Yiwen: 比如说呢？

For example?

[00:06:38.03] Evan: emmmm, 很重要一点就是，这个研究生考虑的这个问题的这个方面和本科生，也不是，这个说什么学历歧视，而是说就是，这个，他们负责的一项工程的这个，不同阶段。emmm, 怎么说呢，比方说这个，他是去写这个底层的代码，而本科生他就只是去用这个封装好的代码，这一点是完全不一样的。然后一方面是从薪资的水平，还有一方面就是，他们做的工作的这个意义，我认为真正去这个顶层去封装这些东西，本质上是没有多大意义的，就是只是去做这个砖瓦匠，这样实际的工作不是很有意义。对。我只，我也不能就是说你，呃，硕士生毕业之后就一定能干这种活儿，只是说它给了你一个门槛，呃不，不叫门槛，叫敲门砖。就是说你至少，理论上，可以和他们，可以和平级的硕士生同起同坐，而不是，领导把你看作本科生，你只能干本科生这样的事儿。所以，工作了一年之后认识到这个本科的学历可能还不够，到最终如果说放弃留学就留在那里工作的话，呃，往上爬的话可能比较吃力。所以最终还是选择这个，工作一年之后就出去留学了。

Emmmm… One important thing is that graduate students see problems from a different perspective than undergraduates. This is not about academic discrimination, but they would be responsible for different stages of a same project. Emm… how to say, for example, the graduate students need to write the underlying code while undergraduates only work with the packaged code, this is completely different. Salary is one thing, but most importantly, it's about the value of your work. As for me, to only work with the packaged code is meaningless. Your work is like a bricklayer. I mean, I just, I cannot guarantee what you can do for sure if you have a master's degree, but it gives you a threshold, uh, no, it's not a threshold, it's a door knocker. That is, you are at least, theoretically, on an equal footing with your co-workers who have master's degree. Otherwise, your leaders would only see you as an undergraduate and assign you the work that undergraduates are supposed to do. So, after working for a year, I realized that a bachelor's degree may not be enough, and if I stay there to work without a master's degree, then, uh, it may be more difficult to get promotions. So, I finally chose to study abroad after working for a year.

[00:08:05.06] Yiwen: 那你在入职的时候你的单位跟你的领导们他们知道你同时还手握一个澳大利亚的学校的 offer，然后你可能会一年之后…

When you entered the company, did they, your leaders know that you were holding an offer from an Australian school in hand, and a year later…

[00:08:12.10] Evan: 是的，是的，我在面试的时候就和他们已经说了，说我可能，只要疫情缓解，我就可能直接"跑路"了。嘿嘿。

Yes, I told them during the interview and said that I might, as soon as the pandemic subsides, I might just "run away". Haha.

[00:08:21.23] Yiwen: 但他们还是…直接录用了你？

But they hired you anyway.

[00:08:22.03] Evan: 对，他们还是要我了，这个就很怪。我也不是，不知道他们怎么想的。是后来，后来事实证明，他们给了一个比较偏的项目，可能就是为了应对我随时"跑路"这种状态。

Yeah, they still hired me, and this was weird. I'm not, I don't know what they were thinking. It was later, and it turned out later, that they gave me a rather marginalized project, probably to deal with the problem t that I might "run away" at any time.

[00:08:34.29] Yiwen: 但是你现在还是在上网课？

And you are still taking online classes now?

[00:08:36.19] Evan: 对，对，是的。我现在还是，是在上网课。

Yes, yes. It's true. I'm still, still taking online classes.

[00:08:39.27] Yiwen: 所以你有没有考虑过，就是暂时不要"跑路"，一边工作一边同时上网课？

So, have you ever considered not "running away" for a while and working while taking online classes at the same time?

[00:08:44.17] Evan: 哎，当时也没有想到这么多。毕竟工作和这个上学，这两种状态是完全不一样的。而且万一这个，在白天，呃出现了，这个重叠的情况，这个时候就不太好处理了。而且我认识到就是，课程的任务还是比较重的，所以我觉得，还是把两者分开来，比较好。当然我认识的同学中也有就是，一边上课一边工作的。但是我认为他们的这样的状态，实在是比较疲劳，而且我本人也不喜欢在 996 之后到家还要上课，这个确实挺累的。

Oops! I didn't think that much. After all, working and taking classes, these two states are completely different. And in case that, in the daytime, uh appear, the time confliction may appear. It can be hard to deal with. And I realize that the task of the course is still relatively heavy, so I think it is better not to do the two things together. Of course, there are students I know who are working while attending classes. But I think they are really tired, and I don't like having classes after working 996[2], which is really tiring.

[00:09:20.12] Yiwen: 你在最开始找工作的时候，你是以为你最终得放弃这个 offer 的，那么到了 2021 年的 7 月份你离职的时候，你当时有想过，要不我就先继续工作着，然后放弃这个 offer，然后直到疫情完全稳定了，我再去上学？有过这种想法吗？

As you mentioned, when you started job seeking, you thought you had to give up the school offer. So, before you left the company in July 2021, have you ever considered keep working till the pandemic end and then reapply for a master's program?

[00:09:40.21] Evan: 肯定有。这个问题其实领导也和我讲过，他也希望能够，呃，边读网课边工作，但是，问题就是，在这个，2020 年这个七月份的时候，疫情还远远看不到结束的时候，对，至少在那个时候（Yiwen: 2021 年 7 月？）啊对对，2021 年 7 月的时候。这个时候，就认识到，如果说再不尽快这个，如果说就是，也不是说尽快，就是，如果你始终是不能去的话，那为什么非要这个纠结于具体哪一年呢？所以，就直接，哪怕先上半年网课，是的，然后再看情况。我是抱着这样的想法。

Of course. In fact, my leader also suggested that I work and take online classes at the same time. The problem was that the pandemic was far from over by July 2020. At least

---

[2] The 996 working hour system (Chinese: 996 工作制) is a work schedule practiced by some companies in the People's Republic of China. It derives its name from its requirement that employees work from 9:00 am to 9:00 pm, 6 days per week; i.e. 72 hours per week. (from Wikipedia: https://en.wikipedia.org/wiki/996_working_hour_system) In Chinese IT companies, the 996 working hour system is very common.

at that moment, (Yiwen: You mean July 2021?) Ah yes, yes, July 2021. At that time, I realized that if I don't go to Australia as soon as possible, I mean, if you are always unable to go, then why obsess about when to go? So, I decided to take online classes for the first half of the year, then find a suitable time to go on site. This is what I thought.

[00:10:32.04] Yiwen: 那么你现在是在"伺机"去澳大利亚 in person 上课吗？

Are you still "waiting for the opportunity" to go to Australia for in-person classes?

[00:10:37.17] Evan: 是的，是的。是"伺机"。但是现在情况是，澳大利亚那边已经似乎已经不把 omicron 当做一回事，但是我心里还是虚的，这毕竟关系到我的身家性命。

Yes, yes. I'm still "waiting for the opportunity." The situation at this moment is that the Australian side seems to have already not taken omicron seriously, but I'm still worried about the pandemic, after all, it is about my own life and health.

[00:10:51.17] Yiwen: 你在做这个决定的时候，你有没有想过你有可能全程网课？

When you were making this decision, did you think about the possibility of you taking all the classes online?

[00:10:55.07] Evan: 哈哈哈哈。这个，这个问题其实，其实挺伤心的。就是，喷，没有，其实我的想法就是至少去一年，但是现在看起来好像只能去半年了。这个，这个，这个其实挺伤心的。哈哈哈。对。其实并没有想过，对。

Hahahaha, it is a sad question. It is, emmm, actually my initial plan was to go on site for at least a year. But now it looks like it can only go for six months. It's such a pity. Hahaha, but I never thought about the possibility of not going to Australia. Never.

[00:11:14.20] (Music)

[00:11:17.12] VoiceOver: 尽管在接受访谈时，Evan还在寻求前往澳大利亚线下上课的时机。我在制作这期播客时，迫于国内互联网行业严峻的就业形势，Evan已经最终放弃了在最后一个学期重返校园的计划，选择留在国内寻找合适的实习机会。Although at the time of the interview, Evan was still "waiting for the opportunity" to travel to Australia to take classes on site. At the time I produced this podcast, Evan had finally given up his plan to return to campus for his final semester due to the tough employment situation in the IT industry in China and decided to stay in China to find an internship.

[00:11:34.16] (Music)

Vol-2 Keke

留学？实习？我都要！硬核武汉女孩的网课生活

Studying Abroad? Internship? I want both! The life of a hard-core Wuhan girl taking online classes

Keke: A master's student majoring in Public Policy at the University of Pennsylvania. She also holds a dual degree in History and International Politics from Peking University. Facing the pandemic, Keke decided to stay in China and take online classes and do some internships at the same time, and eventually completed her post-grad education fully online. As a Wuhaner, she also witnessed the entire process of the pandemic getting worse till the city was locked down for several months and shared those memories with me.

[00:00:00.00] (Music)

[00:00:04.26] VoiceOver: 欢迎来到 The Two Year Stolen，我是 Yiwen。

Welcome to The Two Year Stolen, I'm Yiwen.

[00:00:15.15] VoiceOver: 这一期的受访者是我本科时的同学，Keke，武汉人。她在 2020 年被宾夕法尼亚大学录取，但选择了留在国内，一边上网课一边实习，最终以全程网课的方式完成了自己研究生阶段的全部学业。

The interviewee of this episode is my undergrad classmate, Keke, who is from Wuhan. She was admitted to the University of Pennsylvania in 2020 but chose to stay in China and take online classes and do some internships at the same time. She eventually completed her post-grad education fully online.

[00:00:33.21] (Music)

[00:00:37.11] VoiceOver: 作为武汉人的 Keke，在 2020 年初疫情爆发时，刚刚回到武汉过寒假，于是她见证了武汉疫情渐趋严重，到封城，再到解封的全过程，并与我分享了这段记忆。

Keke, as a Wuhaner, had just returned to Wuhan for winter break when the pandemic broke out in early 2020. She, therefore, witnessed the entire process of the pandemic getting worse till the city was locked down for several months. She shared those memories with me.

[00:00:51.00] Keke: Keke: 我记得武汉当时是，好像是 1 月 23，3 号封的城吧。就是具体的封城日子好像是这一天，然后，嗯，我觉得就是可能我们从封城，在封城的前几天才真正意识到，就是是真的有疫情并且这个疫情它可能很严重，对，所以我是大概 1 月 15 号左右回的，坐火车就放寒假嘛，然后从北京回的武汉。回武汉之后，然后我还很开心地，就约我朋友一起在武汉，就到处吃喝玩乐。然后因为当时也没有意识到疫情就比较严重，所以我们都，就是一开始出了，出门的时候是没有戴口罩的，但是我们看到街上这么多人，当时还是有点害怕。我记得我跟我同学，然后我们当时是在，就是武汉的汉街，然后看到当时街上很多人，我们有点恐慌，我们还是有点怕的，我们就去药店买了两个口罩。

Keke: I remember Wuhan was like, locked down on January 23rd, 23rd. The specific day of the lock-down seemed to be this day. And then, well, I think it was only a few days before the lock-down that we really realized that there was a pandemic and that it could be very serious. Yes. So, I went home around January 15, by train, on winter vacation, from Beijing back to Wuhan. After I returned to Wuhan, I was thrilled to meet my friends in Wuhan, and we hung out and enjoyed ourselves. Then, because we didn't realize that there was a severe pandemic, we all, in the beginning, went out without masks but considering there were so many people on the street, I was a little worried. I remember I was with my classmates, and we were on Han Street,[1] and when we saw many people on the street, we all felt a little panicked and afraid, so we went to the drugstore and bought some masks.

[00:01:50.16] Keke: 而且，那个口罩，嗯，对，我们还是戴上了，但是戴上的时候，像喝奶茶什么的时候我们还是会把它摘掉。然后，那几天其实还并没有说特别的恐慌，真正的恐慌，我觉得大概是封城的前两到三天吧。然后就已经看到新闻里面说可能一下子报道出来好多例，然后并且这个病挺严重的。呃，我记得当时是在，我当时是在那个湖北省图书馆，然后就是可能是在写作业还是干什么，当时好像还要交论文，对，然后看到这个新闻之后，然后当天也提前闭馆了。所有人都，就是很恐慌然后就，就一下子街上面基本上都空了。

Keke: And, that mask, well, yes, we finally put it on, even though, like when we drank bubble tea or something else, we would take it off. The real panic, I think, came about two to three days before the city was locked down. At that time, I saw the news that many cases were reported, and the disease could be quite serious. Uh, I remember being in the, I was in the Hubei Provincial Library at the time. I was probably working on some assignments or so, it seemed like I had to submit an essay at the time, yes, and then after seeing the news, the library closed early that day. Everyone was, was very panicked and then, all of a sudden, the streets were, were almost empty.

[00:02:33.08] Keke: 然后我跟我妈妈，就因为很恐慌，所以我们的本能就是去超市里面，去囤东西。对对对，而且就是让人意外吧，超市里面的人反倒特别特别多。对，然后所有人都在买东西。买完之后可能大概是第二天还是第三天，然后就宣布了封城的消息。

Keke: And then my mother and I, because we were so panicked, our instinct was to go to the supermarket and stock up. And it was a surprise that the supermarket was so crowded. Yes, then everyone was buying things. After this shopping, it was probably the next day or the third day, and then the announcement of the lock-down of the city was made.

[00:02:53.26] Keke: Keke: 我当然其实不是太，不是太敢相信，就是我们真的会封城。因为当时网上已经很多言论说会封城，对，但是我觉得，就因为武汉它本身是个非常重要的交通枢纽嘛，而且当时正值春运，所以说我当时是本（能地），不太相信会封城，但最后，封城的消息出来之后，就感觉大家其实也很快接受了这样的一个事实。

Keke: Of course, I was not too, not too bold to believe that we would really lock down the city. Because at that time, there has been a lot of speculation online that the city would be locked down, yes, but I still thought, because Wuhan itself is a vital transportation hub, and at that time it was the Spring Festival, so I (instinctively) did not quite believe that the city would be locked down. But in the end, after the announcement of the lock-down of the city, it seemed that we actually accepted such a situation quickly.

[00:03:14.15] Keke: 然后整个封城期间，嗯，我其实前期是，前面几天是有点，就是有点兴奋的，说实话。就是，因为我的身边当时还没有遇到就是疫情嘛，就是我

可能我身边的亲戚朋友当时还没有说就是感染上这个病，然后又遇到这么大的一个历史时刻，所以我当时是觉得我可能比如说像见证了这样的一个时刻。

Keke: And then, during the whole period of lock-down, well, I was in the early days, in the first few days, I was a little, was a little excited, to be honest. That is because the people around me were not infected at the time. I mean, my relatives and friends had not yet been infected with this disease, and we were at such a critical historical moment, so I was feeling that I was, like, witnessed such a moment.

[00:03:39.02] Keke: 但是，呃，在2月份的时候，就是这个疫情越来越严重，会发现很多人他已经住不进医院了，然后医疗物资也不够。嗯，大概在2月份的时候，就去报名了那个武汉市红十字会的志愿者，然后担任的是，就是因为武汉市红十字会离我家很近嘛，当时街上面是不允许走那个汽车了，我自己就是可以步行过去，就是上班的。所以我在那里担任志愿者，然后去接听电话。

Keke: But, uh, in February, the pandemic became more and more serious, and we found that many people could not be admitted to the hospital, and then there were not enough medical supplies. Well, in February, I signed up as a volunteer for the Wuhan Red Cross Society, and I worked there because it was very close to my home, and at that time, cars were not allowed on the street, so I was able to walk there and go to work. So, I served as a volunteer there and answered the phone.

[00:04:08.10] Keke: Keke: 对，然后接听电话这个过程我觉得就是见证了，就是，怎么怎么说呢，就是在疫情当中可能不同的人，然后比如说经常会有护士打过来，就是向我们求救那个医疗的物资。我印象特别深的是当时有那个，就是省人民医

院，就是武汉大学附属人民医院的一个护士，给我打电话说他们，他们那边，她是一个消化科的护士，他们那边没有口罩了，就什么也没有，然后就是，感觉所有人都是裸着上去的，对，然后她就向我哭，就是我们告诉她我们这边就是也没有就是分配到他们医院的那个名额，然后最后她就，就是一直在哭，然后我要去安慰她，对。

Keke: Yes, and then answering the phone was a process, I think, it was, I witnessed, how to say, different people's performance in the pandemic. And then, for example, nurses often called us to ask for our help with medical supplies. I was particularly impressed that a nurse from the Provincial People's Hospital, aka the People's Hospital of Wuhan University, called me and said that they had no masks on their side, she was a gastroenterology nurse, they had no masks on their side, they had nothing, and they felt that everyone was exposed to the virus, yes, and then she cried to me. It was, we told her that we didn't have supplies allocated to their hospital. And then she ended up crying, she just kept crying, and then I had to comfort her, yes.

[00:04:49.18] Keke: Keke: 然后接到很多，就是可能外地的一些朋友想要去给我们支援，或者是甚至是想要进来，就是进武汉当志愿者的。就整体还是非常感动吧，这几天。

Keke: Then we got a lot of phone calls, that was, like, some friends from other places wanted to give us support, or even wanted to come in, into Wuhan as volunteers. Overall, I was so moved in those days.

[00:05:02.11] Keke: Keke: 当然这几天我们也经历了网上舆论对于红十字会的一个变化。起因是好像就是寿光给红十字会捐了什么蔬菜之类的，然后说好像我们并没有把它发出去，最后都烂掉了。具体我记不太清了，但是我印象特别深刻的是，在当天上午就是首先是红星新闻，就是国内的红星新闻给我打电话就给，说他是记者然后想要采访我们，然后下午紧接着是新京报，对，但是因为当时红十字会是处于一个，就是红十字会内部它本身这个机构的人员是很少的，就正式工，大量招的都是这种，在疫情的时候大量都是这种志愿者，所以说其实我们人手非常的不足，而且也没有说成立一个专门来应对这种外部舆论的一个专门的就是部门。所以说当时我，我做作为一个志愿者，就是我们志愿者也不知道要把这个电话就是转交给谁，就可能就是在这个当中，就我当时是说，就是我们也没有形成一个官，官方的话术嘛，就所以说我跟那个记者就可能有踢皮球，然后他有可能打给了其他，我们就是红十字会的其他的那个志愿者。

Keke: Of course, in those days, we also experienced a change in online opinions about the Red Cross. It started when Shouguang[2] donated vegetables to the Red Cross, and then it was said that we didn't distribute them out and they ended up decaying. I don't remember in detail, but I was particularly impressed that in the morning, at first, the Red Star News, the domestic Red Star News called me and said he was a journalist and wanted to interview us, and then in the afternoon, followed by the New Beijing News. But because the Red Cross was, that was, the Red Cross itself, the institution's staff is very small, I mean regular workers, a lot of recruitment are, it was, at the time of the pandemic, a large number of volunteers, so we were actually very short-handed, and there was no specific department set up to deal with this kind of external public opinion. So at that time I, I, as a volunteer, was that, we volunteers also did not know whom to pass on these calls. It may be in this period, I was saying, was that we did not formed an official, official words, so that the only thing I could do to the journalist was to pass the buck, and then he may called someone else, I mean other volunteers in the Red Cross.

[00:06:17.00] Keke:最后不知道怎么处理的，但是我看到的就是，这个事情是一个起因，然后之后是更多的人去质疑红十字会，就是他的这样一个，比如他的口罩的分配啊，就各种各种，然后他官僚化，最后在网上是掀起了对于市红十字会和省红十，红十字会的一个骂战。呃，整体来讲的话其实我觉得红十字会是做很多事情的，就是可能网上舆论对他有一些夸张，包括说有一些情绪我觉得这一下子被点燃的那种。对，但是整体来讲确实我感觉就是我们整个，就整个疫情当中是非常的，特别是前期是很慌乱的，就是其实是没有一个非常高效的就是把大家都组织在一起，其实更多是我们志愿者自己去想我们怎么去解决一些事情，对，也没有说给我们一些非常体面或者官方的话术来教我们去应对很多事情。

Keke: I don't know how it was dealt with at last, but what I see is that this issue was a fuse. And then, more people began to question the Red Cross, for, such as the distribution of the masks, and various aspects, and then criticize its bureaucracy. And finally, on the Internet, netizens set off a war of words about the Red Cross of Wuhan and the Red Cross of Hubei Province. Well, overall, I think the Red Cross was doing a lot of things, it is possible that the online public opinions were somehow exaggerated, or emotional. But overall, I do feel that it was very, especially in the early stage, was very disordered. It was, actually, was not so efficient to organize everyone together. In fact, in most situations, it was we volunteers, ourselves to think about how we could solve some problems. And, they did not tell us some very decent or official words to deal with many things.

[00:07:13.14] Keke: 对，然后，嗯，再就是这个志愿服务的同时嘛，就是那几天我就得知我身边的，我高中同学，然后包括最好的姐妹，她就是她的那个，他们的亲人，就是近亲，比如说像妈妈和外公外婆，然后都感染了这个病，对，就是得了这个新冠。嗯，但是他们都没有办法住进医院，就是这个就是在疫情最严重的时候，就是所有人都住不进医院。然后我那个姐妹她的妈妈，是，就是想去请社区的人帮忙然后还去社区去哭闹嘛，因为当时就很绝望，但是也没有办法给她的外婆，就是，甚至没有没有办法给她外婆做检测。就是她的外婆是出现了新冠的症状，但是没有办法确诊，所以最后她的，她外婆也没有住进医院，一直是在家里面自我隔离，然后最后好了。对，但是最后就是疫情结束之后呢，就是稍微也不是结束吧，就是稍微缓解了之后，她外婆去进行了检测，发现是阴性但是体内是有抗体的，对，当时所以就是感觉她应该是那个就是，就是新冠的症状。对。

Keke: Then, well, while volunteering, in those days, I heard that my high school classmates, including my best friend, she was, her, their relatives, close relatives, such as mother and grandparents, were infected with the virus, they got this Covid-19. Well, but they were not able to be admitted to the hospital, that was, that was when the pandemic was at its worst, that was, everyone was not admitted to the hospital. Then my best friend's mother, she, tried to ask the community for help and went to the community to cry. Because at that time it was very desperate, but there was no way to give her grandmother, that was, there was no way to give her grandmother even to be tested. Her grandmother was having symptoms of the Covid-19, but there was no way to confirm the diagnosis, so her grandmother was not admitted to the hospital till the end, and was always at home in self-isolation, and then finally got well. Yes, but finally after the pandemic was over, or I should say it was slightly, not over, it was slightly relieved, her grandmother went for a test and was negative but there were antibodies in her body at that time. So, we believe that she should be, it should be the symptoms of Covid-19.

[00:08:35.26] Keke: Keke: 然后我的姐妹当时是在北京，就不允许回，就他们不让她回武汉。呃，她在北京也很着急，她当时因为我们听说那个爱滋病的药，对是可以治这个新冠的。她当时是在北京市的同志协会去做志愿者，对，因为她是一个就是很关心，然后她当时还就是绝望之下还找了那个北京市同志协会想要给家里面寄一点药。但是那个是就是，很多外面的东西是进，寄，就是没有办法寄到武汉的。最后就这个事就不了了之了。

Keke: Then my best friend was in Beijing at the time. She was not allowed to return, well, they did not let her go back to Wuhan. Uh, she was also very anxious in Beijing, she was then, because we heard that the AIDS medicine was possible to cure this Covid-19. She was volunteering at the Beijing Gay and Lesbian Association, because she was a very caring (person), and then she was also desperate to connect the Beijing Gay and Lesbian Association to mail some medicine to her family. But that was a time, a lot of outside stuff was not, had no way to be mailed to Wuhan. At last, this matter was just left unsettled.

[00:09:10.18] Keke: Keke: 呃，然后我高中同学的话，我高中同学就住在我们家旁边的小区。就我们这个小区是属于老城区，就有很多这种老年人口，所以感染率也是非常得高。然后我高中同学她是，她妈妈，她外公、外婆都感染了，然后都住不进医院。对，嗯，所以，然后知道她，他们，就是她妈妈、外婆都感染之后，她爸连夜把她送到了就是武汉市郊区他们的家里面，就她一个人，在整个封城期间都待在那个家里。对，然后她的爸爸要照，同时照顾她的妈妈还有外公、外婆三个人。然后最后就是她，她当时就很着急，甚至在微博上面去发求助嘛。当时微博上是有很多这个网友去求助，希望自己的亲友能住进医院的。她也尝试去发了，呃，但是效果其实并没有特别的好，甚至会有一些记者吧，就不点名了，就是网上经常骂的某些媒体。

Keke: Well, then my high school classmate, my high school classmate lives in the neighborhood next to our apartment. Our neighborhood is in the old town with a large elderly population, so the infection rate was very high. My high school friend, her mother, her grandfather and grandmother were all infected and could not be admitted to the hospital. Well, so, after knowing that they, aka her mother and grandmother were infected, her father sent her to their another apartment in the suburbs of Wuhan overnight, and she stayed there alone during the whole period of lock-down. Well, then, her father had to take care of her mother, grandfather, and grandmother, the three people, at the same time. Then finally she, she was so anxious, and she even posted messages for help on Weibo.[3] At that time, there were many netizens asking for help on Weibo, hoping their relatives and friends could be admitted to the hospital. She also tried to post something, uh, but the effect was not so good, and even some journalists, I would not say who they were here, but the ones often criticized (for their lack of professional ethics),

[00:10:13.09] Yiwen: 我大概知道！(Laugh)

Yiwen: I think I know who they are!

[00:10:14.18] Keke: 就是有去，有去联系她，说可以帮助她的外公，因为她外公是病得比较严重那种，帮助他的外公就是联系医院，但是是有条件的，就是要接受采访之类的，想要跟她进行这样一个交换。然后她当时就非常的生气，对，然后最后他外公还是住进了医院的，但是她的妈妈，妈妈好像我不知道最后有没有住进医院，对，但是最后的结果还是比较好的，就是三个人都恢复了健康。

Keke: those journalists went to her, went to contact her, saying that they could help her grandfather, because her grandfather was more seriously ill, to help his grandfather reach out to the hospital, but there are conditions, it was to get interviewed or so. They wanted to make such an exchange with her. Then she was very angry, yes, very angry. But at last, his grandfather was admitted to the hospital, but her mother, I do not know if her mother was admitted to the hospital, but the final result was relatively good, that was, all three people recovered.

[00:10:45.17] Keke: 但是有一个事情吧，就是我的那个高中同学，她也是在北京一所高校读书的。呃，当时就是大概是 6 月还是，6 月份的时候，说是毕业生是可以返京，然后参加毕业典礼的。呃，当时她的三个亲人都已经痊愈了，大概是三月份

痊愈的，已经痊愈了三个月了，但是她的辅导员不让她回北京。对，就是，我觉得这个事情其实有点离谱吧，就我们会觉得这个辅导员他可能做的，就是我们，我们其实不太能接受，会感觉到好像他是在，就是在嫌弃我们，或者是他怕担责任。

Keke: But there was another thing. It was that my high school classmate, she is also studying in a college in Beijing. Well, at that time, it was about June or, yes, in June, it was said that the graduates could return to Beijing and then participate in the graduation ceremony. Uh, at that time, all three of her relatives had been cured, probably in March, and had been cured for three months, but her counselor would not let her return to Beijing. Yes, that was, I think this thing was actually a bit ridiculous, we would feel what this counselor did, was, was unacceptable. We would feel as if he was discriminating against us, or he was afraid to take responsibility.

[00:11:26.05] VoiceOver: 而面对"疫情下的留学"这一话题，Keke 告诉我，自己也曾经纠结过是否还要去留学。

When talking about studying abroad during the pandemic, Keke told me that she once had struggled with whether or not to study abroad.

[00:11:34.08] Keke: 就我当时疫情的话，除了为我身边的朋友就是感到非常恐惧，然后去做志愿者，剩下的时间基本上都是躺在家里面，很焦虑。因为当时也是毕业嘛，毕业季，就我不确定我是不是要去留学。当时就很焦虑嘛，觉得自己可能去不了美国，然后就开始在国内找工作。

Keke: At the time of the pandemic, I was very worried for my friends and went to do voluntary work, while the rest of my time was spent at home, anxiously. It was graduation season, and I wasn't sure if I was going to study abroad. At that time, I was very anxious, I thought I might not be able to go to the United States, and then I started to look for a job in China.

[00:11:58.10] Keke: 找工作的时候就发现我还没有做好就是进入职场的准备。就我当时投了很多简历，然后但是我的简历上可能更多都是一些校园的经历，或者是在一些这种公共部门去实习，比如说政府啊，NGO 实习的经历。那我去投企业的话其实并不是特别对口。可能我基本上面试都是靠着我的学校的这种教育背景进的。但是面试的时候会发现我可能对这个部门，或者是业务几乎完全不了解。然后我当时找到的工作都是一些教育机构，就是现在凉掉的那些教育机构。对，就是什么学而思啊之类的，去，就是去当老师。因为我最后面试的时候就会发现，其实好多，就是学校比较好，985 的这种同学，他们最后都会选择去这种教育机构当老师。因为它相对来说门槛比较低，但是它的工资确实还是蛮高的。

Keke: When I was hunting for a job, I realized that I wasn't ready to enter the workplace. I had submitted many resumes at that time, but my resume was probably more about my campus experiences or internships in some public sectors, such as government or NGO. I didn't really match well with the company I was applying to. Maybe I was basically interviewed because of my educational background. But when I was interviewed, I found that I might not know anything about the company or the business. The jobs I found at that time were all in educational institutions. Well, the whole educational industry has been facing great difficulty since 2021. And I got offers from TAL Education Group and some other institutions, and I was about to become a teacher there. And when I was interviewed, I found that, in fact, a lot of students graduated from very good colleges, like project 985 universities,[4] they would choose to work in this kind of educational institution as teachers. Because it is a relatively low threshold with a relatively high salary.

[00:12:55.17] Keke: 然后我当时面临的就是说，我纠结我要不要去这个教育机构先挣一两年钱，然后再去重新申请出国，还是说我就选择网课，就去国外。然后我最后就，我就想着我其实不是特别想，特别喜欢当老师。就是我，我，我，我，我犹豫这个 offer 完全就是因为它钱比较多，就很可能相对来说还比较体面，对。但是我最终还是比较坚持自己内心的想法吧，所以最后把那个当老师的那些 offer 都拒掉了，然后选择了就是在国内以网课的方式来完成了我这个美国研究生的教育。

Keke: Then I was faced with the question of whether I should go to work in an educational institution to earn money for a year or two and then reapply to study abroad, or I should take online classes. Then I ended up thinking that I didn't really want to be a teacher, and I didn't really like it. I was hesitant about this offer only because it paid a lot, and it was probably relatively decent. But I ended up following my heart, so I turned down the offers to become a teacher and chose to complete my graduate education in a school in the United States by taking online classes in China.

[00:13:37.20] Yiwen: 你当时没有考虑过的 defer 一年？

Yiwen: Didn't you consider deferring for a year?

[00:13:40.25] Keke: 我们当时是有，有，有，有向那个院系申请过的。院系当时是允许我们 defer 半年。我当时是想着，就是早一点点毕业，因为我申请的，就是我

申请研究生的一个本（质），最开始其实就是觉得它的学制会稍微短一点，可以稍微早点工作。因为我本身也不是什么学术爱好者。就是我其实最后还是要就业的。那我想着我可能还是早一点工作吧。所以就，当时就没有考虑跟他们一起去 defer 半年。而且说实话，我们那个项目是一年左右，一年左右，即使 defer 半年我也不确定一年半之后我们还能不能去美国，所以我说那我直接我要不就是就还是先，先上着。但是我最后还是选择了延毕，就是我延毕了半年的。所以我实际上跟那些 defer 的同学是一起毕业的。

Keke: We did, did, did, did apply to our department at that time. They allowed us to defer six months. I was thinking, I should graduate earlier because I applied, the reason I applied for a graduate school abroad, at the very beginning was actually that the length of schooling could be a little bit shorter, and I can go to work earlier. Because I myself is not an academic enthusiast. So, I would go to work after graduation. So, I thought I should go to work a little earlier. So, at that time, I did not consider going with them to defer for half a year. And to be honest, our program is about a year, about a year, even if defer half a year, I'm not sure after a year and a half, whether we could go to the United States, so I said that I should take online classes first. But I finally chose to extend for half a year, that was, I graduated six months later than expected. So I actually graduated together with those deferred students.

[00:14:40.28] Yiwen: 你在决定就是要上网课的这个决定的时候，你是对这个疫情什么时候结束有一个大概的预期的吗？

Yiwen: When you made the decision to go online, did you have a general expectation of when the pandemic would end?

[00:14:51.02] Keke: 是国内的还是国外的？

Keke: Domestic or international?

[00:14:52.19] Yiwen: 是有不一样的预期吗？

Yiwen: Did you have different expectations?

[00:14:54.15] Keke: 当时国内的话，国内是好的。就是国内是好了很多的。所以当时我对国内的疫情比较乐观吧，我甚至当时还很傻很天真的，我就想着，因为我面试的时候就是，我那边老师会说话，哇汉武多么多么严重，但是最后会，可能我们这边好转的时候，当时正好是美国最严重的时候。我记得就是2020年大概是下半年，他们那儿就是特别严重嘛，就是大使馆都关了，就不能办签证了。然后我，所以我当时对国内还比较乐观，然后可能我对美国我是持怀疑的态度。对，因为感觉美国那边其实相对来说会比较散养一点嘛，对，我觉得他们那边可能会持续比较（久）。但是我没想到国内会一直，就是一直，就是现在这个样子，就是细水长流的这个，这个样子。

Keke: At that time domestic, domestic was good. In China, it was much better. So, at that time, I was optimistic about the domestic situation, I was even very naïve that I thought, because when I was interviewed, the teachers in UPenn, they would say, wow, you are in Wuhan, the pandemic is so serious there, but in the end, it was like, when the situation here got better, it was the most serious time in the United States. I remember that it was about the second half of 2020, it was so serious there, and even the embassy was closed, you could not apply for the visa. Then I, so I was relatively optimistic about the domestic situation, and then I was probably skeptical about the United States. Yes, because I feel that in the U.S., the policy would be looser. So, I thought the pandemic there would last (longer). But I did not expect the domestic will always, is always, is now like this, round and round.

[00:15:46.11] VoiceOver: 而做出在国内上网课的决定后，Keke 还找到了一份实习，开始了网课和实习并行的生活。

After making the decision of taking online classes in China, Keke also found an internship and began a life of taking online classes and working on the internship at the same time.

[00:15:54.19] Yiwen: 后来你是上网课的同时有找实习，是吗？

Yiwen: Then you did an internship along with your online classes, right?

[00:15:58.08] Keke: 对。我觉得算是因祸得福吧。虽然留学的体验确实挺差的，对，然后跟同学、老师之间的交流可能也没有那么的紧密嘛，相对来说，就甚至是就见不到面嘛也。然后我每次跟我的一些朋友或者是实习的同事就讲，就是我一直在国内上网课的时候，他们甚至会嘲笑我。(Laugh)就是，他们会说，打引号的嘲笑，就是觉得我好可怜。

Keke: Right. I think it's a blessing in disguise. Although the experience of studying was quite bad, and the connections with classmates and teachers may not be so close, relatively speaking, it was not even possible to see each other. Then every time I told some of my friends or colleagues from my internship, they even laughed at me for my stay in China for online classes. (Laugh) That was, they would laugh at, with this laugh at in quotation marks, that they felt sorry for me.

[00:16:29.20] Keke: 对，然后，但是也，也，也是有好处的。就是在国内的话你会离国内的就业的环境是会更近，就是你能真实地感受到国内的那种就业压力，然后也会有更多的时间去，去实习。

Keke: Then, but also, also, there were advantages. If you are in China, you will be closer to the employment environment in China, and you can really feel the employment pressure in China, and then you will have more time to do some internships.

[00:16:46.03] Keke: 我当时，我记得我，我是在字节实习的时候，然后我去交那个，就是交我的在读证明，就是要证明我是一个在校生的身份，就入职的时候。然后我们在排，排队去交的时候，就好多都是在国内上网课的留学生。然后包括我实习的时候我跟我的室友，她是在加拿大的留学生。她本科去加拿大，然后后来又回国了。就是有很多留学生，我会发现很多留学生在国内一边上网课，然后一边去实习。

Keke: I was, I remember I, I was doing an internship in Byte Dance, and then I went to turn in that, that, to turn in my certificate of enrollment, that was, to prove that I was an enrolled student, for entry clearance. When we were in line, there were a lot of international students who were in China for online classes. When I was doing my internship, my roommate and I were working together, and she was an international student in Canada. She went to Canada as an undergraduate, and then returned to China (because of Covid-19). There were a lot of international students, and I found that a lot of international students were taking online classes in China and then going to internships at the same time.

[00:17:19.23] Yiwen: 一边上网课一边实习，累吗？

Yiwen: Was that tiring?

[00:17:23.02] Keke: 非常累。而且我当时是在字节啊，(Yiwen: Laugh) 你知道字节是个什么样的公司！而且我当时还是在字节的创业部门。就整个团队面临的不是说我要做几亿，几亿日活，我们面临的是一个，首先我们要活下去的问题。所以其实是相当于是在字节这样一个大公司内部去做这样一个创业，创业型的产品。我们整个团队的氛围也是一种创业的氛围。有的时候就，我就工作很多，而且非常的 dirty，说实话。然后可能最可怕的是，那几天就有的时候是加班到凌晨。你见过凌晨一点的北京吗？就那种感觉。就是凌晨一两点下班，然后可能跟同事或者室友去吃点东西。然后回家。对，回家之后还要继续就是上网课、写作业。

Keke: It was very tiring. And I was at Byte Dance, (Yiwen: Laugh) you know what kind of company Byte Dance is! And I was even in a startup division of Byte Dance. The whole team was not facing the problem of making hundreds of millions of daily activities, we were facing the problem of surviving first. So, it was actually equivalent to doing such an entrepreneurial product within a big company like Byte Dance. The atmosphere of our whole team was also a kind of entrepreneurial atmosphere. There are times when I work a lot, and it's very dirty, to be honest. And then maybe the worst thing was that there were days when we worked overtime until, until over midnight. Have you ever seen Beijing at 1 am? That was the feeling. It is one or two o'clock in the morning after work, and then maybe with colleagues or roommates, we went for some food. Then we went home. And after you went home, you have to continue to take online classes and writing assignments.

[00:18:15.14] Keke: 我记得我当时就是,我印象特别深刻,就是上了美国的课之后我会发现,一个学分为什么要有这么多东西。就是可能国内的话,就是我们,因为学,就可能也跟我们专业相关吧,就是我们其实没有那么多作业。就可能我们是期中一篇论文,然后期末,期末一个论文一个考,或者一个考试,平时是没有那么多作业要做的。那我就是在这边,就是在美国上课之后发现,每周都要交作业,而且那个作业其实量还挺大的,说实话。就感觉一个学分,就可能一门课只有一个学分,但这个学分真的好难挣啊的感觉。

Keke: I remember I was, what I was particularly impressed, is that after taking the American class, I would feel why there are so many things for one credit! It is possible that back in China, that is, we, or maybe because of the university, or it may also be related to our major, is that we actually did not have so many assignments. It was possible that we had a midterm essay and then at the end of the semester, another essay, or an examination. Usually, we didn't have so many assignments. However, here, I found that I had to turn in assignments every week, and the workload was actually quite large, to be honest. I feel that only one credit, it may be for one course, only accounts for one credit, but this credit is really hard to earn.

[00:18:51.07] Keke: 然后我基本上每天下班回家,然后别人,就我室友都已经躺在床上,开一局王者,或者是就直接睡着了,在那边打呼了,然后我在这边还要写作

业。我经常写着写着我就觉得自己为什么这么惨。然后就有时候就写着写着睡着了，然后我就在桌子上面趴了一晚上，第二天起来，发现作业没有写完，然后还要去上班。就是这个样子。那段时间说实话还蛮痛苦的。

Keke: Then basically every day after I came home from work, when my roommate has been lying in bed, playing Honor of Kings,[5] or she just fell asleep, snoring over there, and then I had to write assignments. I often wrote and wrote, and I thought why I was so miserable. Then sometimes I fell asleep while writing, and I slept at my desk all night. Then the next day, I got up and found that I had not finished my assignment, and then I had to go to work. That's how it was. That time was quite painful, to be honest.

[00:19:20.26] Yiwen: 那你们会有上课的时间和你上班的时间冲突的情况吗？

Yiwen: And did you have any time conflict between your classes and your work?

[00:19:26.26] Keke: 会有。因为那边的课基本上都是国内时间的晚上。所以我经常面临的就是，要一边加班然后一边上网课。所以我当时主要是在，就是这边工作着，然后那边就把那个课程挂在，就是挂着嘛。然后有个时候会被，也会被 leader 发现，他会问你在干什么。但是因为我同事其实都知道我在上网课，因为他们都分别地嘲笑过我，所以其实也还好。(Laugh)

Keke: There would be. Because the classes were basically at night during the domestic time. So, I was often faced with having to work late and having online classes at the same time. So, I was mainly doing my work and kept online for the classes, I had to keep online. Then sometimes my leader would find that I was taking classes, then he would ask what I was doing. But because all my colleagues actually knew that I was taking online classes, because they all separately laughed at me, so, it was actually okay.

[00:19:57.08] Yiwen: 那会一心二用？

Yiwen: So it was like dual-tasking?

[00:19:58.26] Keke: 当然没有啦！主要的精力都还是在听课，因为工作还是可以摸鱼的嘛，(Laugh) 就我只要正常把任务交了，摸个鱼什么的，反正我 leader 也不会 care，对。

Keke: Of course not! My main focus was listening to the class, because I could mess around at work. (Laugh) As long as I could hand in the tasks in time, my leader would not care anyway.

[00:20:13.02] Yiwen: 但是这样可能就要加班加更长时间？

Yiwen: Then you may have to work overtime longer?

[00:20:16.03] Keke: 对，这个确实是。就是有时候可能下班更晚，或者说要把工作带回去做。天呐！那几个月我经历了什么！(Laugh) 我现在回想我觉得好恐怖啊！就真的就是睡眠不足！

Keke: Yes, this is true. It was that sometimes you had to get off work even later or take work home. Gosh! What I went through in those months! (Laugh) When I look back on it now, I feel it's horrible! Really lack of sleep!

[00:20:29.09] (Music)

Vol-3 71

赴美半年后遭染新冠肺炎，哥大女生分享自己遭染前后的心路历程

Columbia student shares her story of getting Covid-19 after arriving in the U.S. for half a year

71: A master's student in the East Asian Languages and Cultures Program at Columbia University. Before entering Columbia University, she majored in Biological Science and Chinese Literature at Peking University. 71 had a gap year because she didn't want to take online classes. Right before the winter break in 2021, she unexpectedly tested positive for Covid-19, which she didn't dare to tell her family.

[00:00:00.00] (Music)

[00:00:04.26] VoiceOver: 欢迎来到 The Two Year Stolen，我是 Yiwen。

Welcome to The Two Year Stolen, I'm Yiwen.

[00:00:15.12] VoiceOver: 这一期的受访者是我在哥大时的好朋友，71，本科毕业于北京大学。

The interviewee of this episode is my friend at Columbia, 71, who graduated from Peking University as an undergraduate.

[00:00:21.16] (Music)

[00:00:24.04] VoiceOver: 疫情爆发的时候，71 正值大四。因为疫情，学校不断地推迟开学，她的毕业设计也受了一些影响。

71 was in her senior year when the pandemic outbroke. The school kept postponing the start of the new semester because of the pandemic, and her plan for the final project was also disrupted.

[00:00:32.15] 71: 一开始爆发的时候，应该是在我大四上的时候，当时应该是寒假已经回家了。我当时没有预料到它会这么严重。我当时是觉得我可能过完一个春节，我就又可以重返我的学校了。呃，所以后来学校有发布延迟开学的消息，我有一些惊讶，但是我觉得可能延迟一个月开学，可能我又可以回去了，但是一直不断地延迟，我没有想到最后我的毕业设计也是在家里完成的。

The pandemic outbroke when I was in my senior year. It should be in the winter break, and I have already gone home for holiday. I didn't anticipate it would be this serious at the time. I was thinking that I might be able to go back to my school right after the Spring Festival. Uh, so when there was an announcement of a later start of the new semester, and I was shocked. But I thought maybe a month of postponing would be enough, and I could go back to campus after a month. But it kept postponing, and I didn't think I would end up finishing my final project totally at home.

[00:01:09.11] Yiwen: 整个在家完成毕业设计的过程当中，有因为在家导致毕业设计遇到一些麻烦吗？

Have you met any problems when you worked on your final project at home?

[00:01:17.02] 71: 有的。因为我其实当时的毕业设计是必须要在实验室完成的一些实验，就是因为我无法返回学校，包括我在内，还有很多学生，最后我们的选择都是用生物信息学的方法去完成最后的毕业论文。

Sure. Actually, according to my initial plan, I had to complete some experiments in the lab. However, I could not go back to the campus. Many students, including me, had to finish our final project with Bioinformatics approaches.

[00:01:35.24] Yiwen: 所以这个是（相当于）整个你的毕业设计的方向就转向了。
Does this mean that the whole direction of your final project has changed?

[00:01:41.12] 71: 对，这就是整个方法需要改变。因为我不能到实验室了，所以可能需要重新学一些软件，但是课题基本上没有太大的变化。但是我觉得这个也不能说是一件坏事，因为我觉得，因为首先，如果我重返校园，我其实上也只剩下最后一个学期的时间去给我做实验，其实对于完成毕业论文来说，也是时间上还是有一点紧张。如果在家的话，我可以利用自己的时间去学一门新的程序，或者新的软件，去做一个毕业设计，我觉得这也不是一件特别糟糕的事情。

Yes, I had to change the whole methodology. Since I could not go back to the lab, I had to learn some new software from the beginning. But the subject itself has not changed much. But I don't think this is a bad thing, because I think, first, if I went back to campus, I could have only one semester to do all the experiments, which was not enough for my thesis. But I stayed at home, and I could use more time to learn new software and finish my project, which might be better.

[00:02:21.21] VoiceOver: 71 从大三开始准备出国留学的相关事宜，到疫情爆发的时候，她其实已经得到了一些 offer。并且，随着美国的疫情越来越严重，在发现自己无法在 2020 年赴美之后，71 最终选择了延期一年入学。

71 began to prepare for studying abroad in junior year and had already received some offers when the pandemic outbroke. However, as the situation in the U.S. got worse, 71 eventually chose to defer for a year after she realized she would not be able to come to the U.S. in 2020.

[00:02:39.17] 71: 应该是在大三的时候。我当时是在跨院保研和出国留学之间做选择。我当时想，如果不能跨院保研的话，我就出国留学。这两条路我是同时进行的。

I think I started preparing in my junior year. At that time, I had a choice between applying for a graduate program in another department at PKU and studying abroad. I thought if I could not enter the Chinese Literature department at PKU, I would study abroad. I prepared for both at the same time.

[00:02:58.12] Yiwen: 后来因为没有能够？

Then you weren't able to…

[00:03:01.04] 71: 对，因为没有能够成功的跨院保研，我就想，那就出国吧。因为我其实出国的一些准备我都已经都完成了。

Yes. I failed in applying for the graduate program in the Chinese Literature department and I thought, 'OK, fine, let me study abroad.' And I have already finished all the preparation for applying for graduate school abroad.

[00:03:10.10] Yiwen: 就是语言考试这些？

Like language tests?

[00:03:12.12] 71: 对。都同时进行，所以我就没有太多的顾虑。

Yes. I prepared simultaneously. So I didn't have too much worry.

[00:03:17.10] Yiwen: 那差不多当疫情爆发的时候，你的这些申请都已经提交出去了。

So when the pandemic broke out, you have already submitted all the applications?

[00:03:21.10] 71: 对。当时已经，对，都已经提交出去。

Yes. I have submitted them all.

[00:03:23.02] Yiwen: 属于一个在等待他们给你发 offer 的阶段？

And you were waiting for offers?

[00:03:27.07] 71: 甚至已经有 offer 了。

Yes. And I have even received some.

[00:03:28.12] Yiwen: 疫情爆发的时候？

When the pandemic outbroke?

[00:03:28.12] 71: 对，但只是口头的。对。

Yes. Though only oral offers. Yes.

[00:03:32.21] Yiwen: 所以你当时有想过疫情可能会影响到你出国留学的计划吗？

So have you thought the pandemic might influence your plan to study abroad at that time?

[00:03:38.10] 71: 我当时没有想过。因为当时主要是在中国爆发，我没有想到，

（[00:03:45.09] Yiwen: 没有想到它会）对，会蔓延到我想要去的留学的国家。

Absolutely not. Cuz the pandemic was happening mainly in China, and I didn't anticipate (Yiwen: you didn't anticipate it would…) yes, it would spread to the country I would like to go.

[00:03:48.22] Yiwen: 美国这边大概是三、四月份的时候就开始有疫情，那个时候你有开始担心自己可能暂时去不了美国吗？

The pandemic broke out in the United States around March or April. At that time did you start to worry that you might not be able to go to the U.S. for a while?

[00:03:57.12] 71: 我其实到三、四月份的时候我都没有太担心。因为我还是觉得可能国内的情况会比国外更严重。我选择去国外留学，其实并不会受到太大的阻碍。

In fact, I wasn't too worried until March or April. Because I still thought that maybe the situation would be worse at home than abroad. My plan to study abroad would not really be influenced too much.

[00:04:07.14] Yiwen: 你最后还是选择 defer 一年。 defer 决定是在什么时候做出来的？

However, you still chose to defer for a year at last. So, when did you make that choice?

[00:04:11.05] 71: 具体的时间我忘记了，但是大概是，应该是我知道了美国的疫情已经严重到可能对我出入境可能会有影响的时候。

I forget the exact time, but it was probably, I think when I learned that the pandemic in the US had become so serious that it might have had an impact on my entry.

[00:04:24.01] Yiwen: defer 的一年，你主要在家都做些什么？

What did you do during the year?

[00:04:27.07] 71: 毕业之后的暑假是在家里待着的。在开学的时候我又去到北京，我在北京跟一个朋友一起合租。然后当时有去学校听课什么的。对，继续听课。

I stayed at home during the summer holiday after graduation and went back to Beijing after the holiday. I rented an apartment with a friend in Beijing. I sometimes would go back to the college and audit some classes. Yes, I kept going to school.

[00:04:44.11] Yiwen: 那时候已经毕业的学生也可以进去（学校）？

Students who had already graduated could also enter the campus at that time?

[00:04:46.22] 71: 当时是我当时的老师，他说我可以过去跟他见个面，但是其实北大管得比较严，所以不太好进去，但是清华是可以进去的，所以我有在清华里面听一些课。

It was my professor. He told me to see him on campus. In fact, the policy to access the campus in PKU was relatively strict and it was hard to get into PKU. However, it's easier to get into Tsinghua and I audited some classes there.

[00:05:01.14] Yiwen: 大概一些什么样的课？

Like what?

[00:05:02.19] 71: 各个系的吧。社会学系、历史学系、还有应该是他们的外文系吗？我不太清楚是什么系开的课，反正听了一些课。

Classes in various departments. Sociology department, history department, and I think it's their foreign language department? I'm not quite sure what departments offered the classes, but I audited some of them anyway.

[00:05:12.23] VoiceOver: 在 71 看来，defer 是她在当时可以做出的最优的选项。

In 71' eyes, deferring for a year was the best choice she could made at that moment.

[00:05:16.29] 71: 因为当时我们的情况，如果你不 defer 的话，你就得在家上网课。我有问过我一些上网课的同学，基本上他们那种昼夜颠倒的作息，我觉得对他们进行这一年的学习，我觉得也是不太好的。就比如他们可能都是在凌晨上课，脑子极度不清醒，课堂参与也非常不积极，和老师的互动也不够多，跟同学也不能建

立一个比较紧密的关系，所以会让我觉得你花了很高的成本去上一个非常没有真实感的学吧。

I was facing a situation where if I didn't defer, I had to have online classes at home for a whole year. I asked some of my friends who chose to have online classes afterward and I felt their day and night inversion life would influence their studies. Like they had to enter classes at midnight and their mind was not clear enough. They could not participate in class actively, have enough interaction with the professors, and establish close relationship with their classmates. It would make me feel like paying a lot to attend a graduate program that lacks a real sense.

[00:05:54.19] VoiceOver: 到了 2021 年，已经延期一年入学的 71，与自己的父母在是否需要赴美这件事情上依旧存在着分歧。

Until 2021, even after a gap year, 71 still have some different ideas with her parents over whether or not to go to the US.

[00:06:02.11] 71: 父母会不断的每天会暗示你，可能会告诉你现在国外的疫情如何如何，如果是这样，你还要去吗？可能每天都会问一句。对，他们通过这种问话不断会让你明白，其实可能你有可能你真的去不了了。但是同时你心里又有个声音想要反驳他们，没有那么严重，可能只是你们家长的想法对吧，最终我们还是可以去的。所以到最后我家长可能会这样说，他觉得我可能是出去读书不要命的。

（[00:06:39.04] Yiwen: 哈哈哈哈。）（笑）他会有这样的一种说法。

My parents would constantly imply to me by telling me how the situation was abroad right now and asking if I insisted on going. They would ask me every day. Yes, through this kind of questioning they would constantly make me understand that maybe I really could not go. But at the same time, there was a voice in my heart that I wanted to counter them that it wasn't that serious, that it was probably just their ideas, and I could eventually go. So, my parents would sometimes joke that I could even give up my life to study abroad. ([00:06:39.04] Yiwen: Hahahahaha.) (Laughs) They would have that kind of argument.

[00:06:41.12] Yiwen: 所以你的父母其实是到后来不是特别的支持你出来？

So your parents were actually not really supportive of you coming to the U.S.?

[00:06:45.11] 71: 对。但是他们又没有非常强硬地反对，他们只是通过一种言语暗示告诉你它的风险在哪里。我的方式也是用一种开玩笑的方式，但是也非常认真地告诉他们，其实没有你们想得那么严重。我会不断地拿数据来告诉他们，我会习惯性的把可怕的数据不告诉他们，把有一些积极的信息，比如疫情已经有在好转了，或者有什么研发出来的（Yiwen：疫苗。）对，有一些什么利好的消息，我会每天都会告诉他们。对，但是他们是他们是不太相信的。

Yes. But they didn't really oppose it strongly either, they just told you where the risks were by implication. And I also argued in a joking way, though seriously, by telling them that it was not as serious as they thought. I would keep convincing them with data, I would habitually hide the scary data and give them positive information like the situation is getting better, or scientists have made some progress (Yiwen: like a vaccine.) Yes, when there was some good news, I would tell them. But they didn't really believe it.

[00:07:27.21] Yiwen: 当你最后真正你可以出来的时候，他们也就没有再反对了？

But when you could finally come to the U.S., they stopped objecting?

[00:07:32.09] 71: 他们其实一直都没有在太反对。他们只是觉得，我需要意识到，你有可能出不去，你要想好你接下来要做什么。他只是在做一个提醒吧，如果最后我能出去，他们当然是很开心的。对。

They haven't actually been too opposed to it. They just thought that I needed to be aware that there was a chance that I wouldn't go to the U.S., and I had to figure out what I was going to do then. I was just a reminder. They were definitely happy when I was able to come to the U.S.

[00:07:48.09] Yiwen: 那你当时有按照他们所说的去做一个，比如说，如果出不去的 plan b 吗？

So did you follow what they said to make a, for example, plan B?

[00:07:53.19] 71: 没有，完全没有。

No, never.

[00:07:54.29] Yiwen: 你觉得我肯定是可以出去的？（71:对。）如果你想象一下，如果在 2021 年的时候，你在现实生活中你是确实能过来的，但如果你当时没有能够过来。（71:对。）你在那个时候你会是再等一年还是再去想别的办法？

You were convinced that you could come? (71: Yes.) So let us imagine, in 2021, if, I mean, in the reality, you could come to the U.S., but if you couldn't, would you defer for another year or make another choice?

[00:08:14.21] 71: 如果一年之后还是，如果我 gap 一年之后还是不能过去，我就选择上网课，因为我不可能推迟两年。对，而且我的项目也不允许推迟两年。

If after the gap year, I still could not come, I would have online classes. It's impossible for me to defer for two years, and it's not allowed by the program.

[00:08:26.18] Yiwen: 所以其实你还是有考虑过如果出不来的话我要怎么办的?

So, you still had a plan B?

[00:08:32.26] 71: 对。但是这个不是我考虑的问题,就是如果一年我还是出不来,我只能被迫上网课。这是被动的一个选择。对。

Yes, but it was not about my choice. I was forced to take online classes. That's completely passive.

[00:08:42.27] VoiceOver: 刚到美国的时候,对于新冠疫情,71 采取了非常谨慎的态度。

When she first arrived in the United States, 71 took a very cautious attitude to the pandemic.

[00:08:47.27] 71: 我有个朋友,她约我去宜家逛一下,然后我当时问了一下我父母可不可以去,我父母是强烈反对,(笑)因为他觉得如果我去,可能要坐地铁上,人比较多,暴露的风险也比较高。

I have a friend. She invited me to go to IKEA with her. And I asked my parents whether I could go and they strongly opposed it. (Laugh.) They believe that going to IKEA means taking the subway while taking the subway means exposure to viruses.

[00:09:03.25] Yiwen: 那后来你是什么时候开始,可能没有那么的在乎你父母的意见,开始出门堂食呀,还有出去逛街呀这些?

Then when did you start to care less about your parents' opinions and start going out for dinners and shopping?

[00:09:13.00] 71: 我觉得这个可能是因为我上课的原因，就是我有一节课，一周是要出去上4次的一门语言课。当时每次上完课之后，同学们都会说，大家要不要一起吃饭。这种情况下，你不可能再用一种觉得出去吃饭危险，很危险这种理由去搪（塞），也不是搪塞或者去不接受，这样子会显得你特别不合群。对，所以可能你也答应了一次。之后可能就习惯了跟同学一起吃饭。如果你一开始你能接受在食堂里堂食，那慢慢你就可以接受在外面的餐厅开始吃东西，慢慢的你朋友约你外出，你可能也就也就可以认，也就会同意了。

I think it was because of a class I took. I was taking a language class in which I had to attend class 4 times a week outside the campus. Every time after class, some classmates would suggest going out for lunch together. In this situation, it's not possible to give the runaround for the reason that it's dangerous to dine in. This would make me look very asocial. So I joined them for the first time. After that, I got used to eating with my classmates. And if you can accept to eat in the cafeteria at first, then slowly you can accept to go to a restaurant. Gradually, you may accept going anywhere.

[00:10:01.04] Yiwen: 所以其实最开始是为了合群？

So at first it was about fitting in?

[00:10:03.01] 71: 对，一开始是为了合群，因为当时周围人的态度并没有把这个看作一件很可怕的事情。如果你特别的恐惧的话，其实会显得有点奇怪。

Yes. It was about fitting in. Because people around me didn't see it as a very scary thing. It would seem to be a bit wield if I performed so restless.

[00:10:17.04] VoiceOver: 在逐渐放松警惕之后不久，71 发现自己感染了新冠病毒。

Shortly after lowering her guard, 71 found herself infected with the coronavirus.

[00:10:23.11] Yiwen: 你在去年冬天的时候其实是感染过一次新冠的？（71: 嗯。）能跟我们讲讲当时的情况吗？

You once got Covid last winter? (71: Yes.) Could you briefly talk about the situation at that time?

[00:10:29.29] 71: 因为当时放了一个 3 天的短假，我和同学去了一趟费城。（Yiwen: 感恩节？）应该是感恩节，对。然后我和同学去了一趟费城，当时我觉当时我其实已经放松警惕了吧，我可以说。就是我只是戴上了口罩，我就觉得自己做好了防护，但是我内心的那种防护意识，我觉得已经完全松懈下去了。所以我猜想可能在费城，在餐厅堂食的时候可能更被感染了。

I took a trip to Philadelphia with my friends because we had a 3-day vacation. (Yiwen: Thanksgiving?) I think it was Thanksgiving. And I went to Philadelphia with my friends, and I have to say I was not so cautious. I just put on my mask, and I felt like I was protected, but my consciousness loosened up. So I guess I might get infected in Philadelphia when dining in a restaurant.

[00:10:58.19] Yiwen: 你是什么时候意识到自己可能感染的？

When did you realize that?

[00:11:01.02] 71: 我其实一直都没有觉得自己可能感染了。我更多的是出一种怕自己感染会传染到别人，这样这件事情的影响就会非常不好。我从来都没有觉得自己会感染，对。我只是通过去检测来排除别人对我的一种疑惑吧，或者就是那种恐惧。因为当时我有感冒，其实我，跟我一上课的同学就会很明显发现你说话有鼻音啊，或者你有感冒的症状，他们可能不会有明显的恐惧，但是心里会有一些担忧。这时候我只是想去测一下，通过这个结果，我告诉他们我没有得，对，这样他们可以继续跟我一起愉快地吃饭。对，我当时的想法是这样子。

I actually never thought I might be infected. I was more out of a fear that I might infect others so that the impact of this thing would be very bad. I never felt like I was infected, yes. I just did the test to reduce others' doubts, or maybe fears, about me. Because I had symptoms of a cold at the time. My classmates could easily find my nasal voice. They might not show it, but you could feel that they had some concerns about staying with you. At this point, I just wanted to do a test to prove I didn't get covid. In this way they could continue to have fun with me without any worries. That's what I was thinking.

[00:11:48.17] Yiwen: 你觉得我自己并没有感染，我就是普通的流感？（71: 对。）然后我必须得去做一个核酸检测，用事实说话。

You believed it was not Covid but flu? (71: Yes.) And you felt you had to do a test and prove your "innocence" with the result?

[00:11:59.15] 71: 对，而且，但是我还是想如果真的感染了，我还是早发现，尽量减少我给别人带来的影响。

Yes. And if I really got Covid, finding it earlier would be better for I would influence fewer people.

[00:12:07.11] Yiwen: 你是从费城回来之后大概多久去做的核酸？

When did you do the test? How many days after you came back from Philadelphia?

[00:12:11.08] 71: 费城回来3天后。对。应该是3天后，我记得不太清楚了。

3 days after coming back. Yes, I think it should be 3 days later. I cannot remember clearly.

[00:12:19.09] Yiwen: 因为你自己没有觉得你自己感染了，所以在那之前你其实是跟朋友正常社交的？

Considering you didn't think you got covid, were you and your friends still socializing normally before you tested positive?

[00:12:25.17] 71: 因为费城回来的时候我整个人感觉非常得疲惫，我当时以为是旅行给我带来的。因为当时睡眠不太好，一天的行程也我觉得非常累，我当时应该旅行完，在家当感觉应该是躺了有一天吧。我当时觉得我累了，但是后来就慢慢发现自己头非常的痛，可能有一些发烧的症状吧。主要是和我，和我在一起的另一个朋友也出现了这种症状，她也建议我要去测一下，她觉得她自己要去测一下。我当时约了能约到最早的一次。它一般来说，它会是通过邮件发一个实验室的结果报告，通过邮件的形式发给你。当时我一直没有收到邮件，其实我心里就觉得有一点不对劲了。到下午的时候，而且当时我收到结果的当天中午，我还跟朋友一起饭。

When I came back from Philadelphia, I felt very tired, which I thought was caused by the trip. Because I didn't sleep well, and the one-day trip was really tiring. I should have stayed in bed for a whole day after the trip. I thought I was tired, but then I found myself having a very bad headache and probably a fever. And a friend who went to Philadelphia with me also had these symptoms. She went for a test and suggested that I should also do a test. I made the earliest appointment I could get. Usually, you would receive a result report from the lab by email in one day. When I did not receive this email in time, I felt that there might be a problem. But right before I received the results, I still had lunch with my friends.

[00:13:17.09] Yiwen: 对，你那天还约我，我们俩还约饭了。（笑）

Yes, you invited me for lunch that day.

[00:13:19.09] 71: 对对对，我当时遇到你。（笑）对，当时我课友正好又在一起吃饭，所以我当时好像最后也没有跟你一起吃饭。（Yiwen: 对。）后来回去的时候，我在家里休息的时候，我就接到了一个陌生的电话，我当时就觉得有点不太对劲。然后我拿起电话，对方就说很抱歉你的结果是阳性。（笑）

Yes. When I met you in the cafeteria, I was having lunch with my classmate. But I didn't have lunch with you at last. (Yiwen: Yes.) Then after lunch, I was having a rest at home, and I got a call from a stranger. I felt there might be some problem but still answered the call. The guy gold me, "Sorry, your test result is positive." (Laugh)

[00:13:42.06] Yiwen: 你就开始自我隔离？

Then you began the self-quarantine?

[00:13:43.14] 71: 他当时是说，他当时告诉我这个结果，他就说你现在要避免见他人，可以自我隔离。然后有什么需要注意的，他过一会晚上还会再给我打一个电话。

He told me the result and asked me to avoid seeing any other people and suggested a self-quarantine. And he told me he would call back at night to give me more detailed notes.

[00:13:57.19] Yiwen: 他晚上又给你打了一个电话？

So he called back at night?

[00:13:59.04] 71: 对，他晚上又给我打电话，询问我的症状，然后告诉我应该做什么。我觉得他说的不是很详细，我觉得他的核心意思就是我只要去做好自我隔离就可以了。甚至他也没有，没提醒我。我可以跟我的密接说一下，他们也需要做一个检测。但是我事后知道好像我们学校是会有一个追踪你密接的一个流程的。

Yes, he called me again at night and asked about my symptoms and then told me what I should do. I don't think he was very detailed, I think the core of what he was saying was that I should have a self-quarantine. And he even didn't, didn't tell me that I could tell my close contacts and they might need a test. But I know afterward that our school seems to have a process for tracking close contacts.

[00:14:20.14] Yiwen: 那我应该就没有被算在你的密接里面，所以我没有被追踪到。因为我们那天只是打了个招呼，你没有跟我一起吃饭。

I shouldn't have been counted as your close contact, so I wasn't tracked. Because we just said hi that day but not having lunch together.

[00:14:27.11] 71: 对对对，应该可能就没有算进去。

Yes. You might not have been counted.

[00:14:29.05] Yiwen: 对,但是你通知了我,所以我去做了检测。学校有给你发一些什么…

But you informed me, and I had a test. Did the school send you any…

[00:14:32.25] 71: 他给我发了一个急救包,急救包,但是是在我已经好了的时候他才送到。(笑)

They sent me a first aid kit. But the package was sent to my home after I had recovered. (Laugh.)

[00:14:38.18] Yiwen: 所以你在自我隔离的时候,你有自己去想一些办法来…

So during the self-quarantine, did you find some way to…

[00:14:43.24] 71: 自救是吗?(Yiwen: 对。)我当时觉我需要提高我的免疫力,所以我当时休息会睡得比平时会早一些。然后在饮食上,我会比平时摄入更多的蛋白质。(笑)我还去网上买了各种维生素,什么(Yiwen: VC之类的?)对 VC 还有锌片。对,各种药。

Self-aid? (Yiwen: Yes.) I felt like I needed to enhance my immunity, so I slept earlier than usual. And in terms of diet, I would eat more protein, (laughs) and I bought all kinds of vitamins online, like (Yiwen: VC?) yes, VC and zinc tablets, all kinds of medicines.

[00:15:15.08] Yiwen: 也不是药,就是保健品?(笑)

Not really medicines but supplements?

[00:15:17.00] 71: 对,保健品。药也买了。对。

Yes, supplement. I also bought some medicines.

[00:15:20.14] Yiwen: 药买的是连花清瘟？（71: 连花清瘟。（笑））

I guess you bought Lianhua Qingwen Capsule? (71: Yes, Lianhua Qingwen Capsule. (Laugh))

[00:15:20.14] Yiwen: 他们也没有提示你，美国这边一般大家都吃什么药？

Didn't they tell you what people in the U.S. usually take for treatment?

[00:15:25.15] 71: 他说如果我有感（冒），发烧的症状，他说我可以去买退烧药，但是我整个患病的过程我就没有发过特别高的烧。通常情况我觉得如果是低烧，我基本上是我是可以不吃药，它烧就能退的。

He said that if I had a cold and a fever, I could take some antipyretic, but I haven't had a particularly high fever the whole time I've been sick. Usually, I think if it was a low fever, basically no need to take medicine.

[00:15:42.05] Yiwen: 所以其实你的症状不是很严重？

So your symptoms were not so serious?

[00:15:44.08] 71: 对。

Yes.

[00:15:45.01] Yiwen: 大概多久之后你痊愈了？

About how long did it take for you to recover?

[00:15:48.19] 71: 如果以它最后转阴为标准，我觉得一个月吧，我记得是。

I think a month if you mean my test result turned negative.

[00:15:56.04] Yiwen: 是从出现症状开始？

Counted from the emergence of symptoms?

[00:16:00.16] 71: 对，到转阴。因为我当时其实患病的时候是在我期末季，我当时已经把寒假的行程都已经安排好了，所以我突然被这个感染嘛，取消了所有的计划。我当时其实是想我希望我快一点再去检测，快点证明我转阴了，这样我又可以跟我的朋友继续出去玩。我当时，所以我特别急。我基本上我当时是想一周测两次，因为我当时有查到消息，有些人可能一周就可以转阴。我当时就想自己也可能抵抗力比较好，说不定可以这么快就能转阴。所以我当时一周就想测两次。一开始的时候是可以的。后来应该是我去第三次的时候吧，一直都没有转阴，第三次去测的时候，当时学校就告诉我说你不能这么频繁地测，他还发了一个邮件告诉我，如果已经测出有阳性的人，他可能未来大概 90 天内都不需要再测。

Yes, and till I tested negative. Because I got sick in the final week, and I had already arranged my winter break trip. I had to cancel all my plans. And I wanted to get tested again soon to prove that I had recovered, so I could travel with my friends again. I was, so I was anxious. At first, I wanted to test twice a week, because I had heard that some people could turn negative in only one week. I thought I had good physical qualities, so I might be able to turn negative very quickly. I went to do the test twice a week. I was allowed to do so at the very beginning, but when I went there for the third time, my test result was still positive, and the staff told me that I should not test so often. He even sent me an email telling me that if someone has already tested positive, he may not need to test again for the next 90 days or so.

[00:17:01.26] Yiwen: 所以你后来就没有再频繁地去做检测。然后大概过了一个月你去测，你已经阴了？

So you didn't go back for a test till a month later, and you were finally negative?

[00:17:10.02] 71: 对，因为其实你每次测的，也挺让你的心态挺崩溃的。因为你觉得你，因为我的症状来说，我自己觉得已经完全好了，但是它结果来看，你确实没有转阴，但其实你可其实已经是没有不具备传染性的。但是如果你想要跟别人一起出去，你不可能跟别人说我现在还是阳性，但我已经没有传染性了，这种话你只有自己会，自己可以这样说服自己嘛。所以学校就算，他不是让我90天内不去测，我还是又约了，只不过我的频率不可能每周两次，我大概两（周），十天一次吧，我可能还是测。最后我记得应该，应该是我去测的第五次就变成阴了，我记得。

Yes, because it can be quite annoying that you went to do a test with high expectations but could never get the results you wanted. According to the symptoms, I felt I have already recovered, but the test result was still positive. Though you knew the virus was no longer infectious to others, if you wanted to hang out with someone, you could not tell them that your test result was positive, but they were safe. This can only be used for self-assurance. So even though my doctor told me not to get tested for 90 days, I made another appointment. I just went less frequently, from twice a week to once every two weeks or ten days. And it should be the 5th time I went for a test, I finally turned negative.

[00:17:58.12] Yiwen: 然后阴了你就终于松了口气？

Then you got some kind of relief?

[00:18:00.18] 71: 对，而且还有一件事情是，原来跟我一起准备去寒假一起旅游的那个同学，她寒假的时候也一直没有联系我，当时觉得特别奇怪，后来我，我当时在，也偶然知道她也阳性了。

Yes. And another thing is about the friend with whom I was preparing to travel together during winter break. She didn't contact me during the whole winter break. I felt strange at first, and then I happened to know that she also tested positive.

[00:18:21.13] Yiwen: 所以你们两个本来要一起去旅游。最后…

So you initially planned to go for a trip together but end up…

[00:18:23.29] 71: 对，双双阳性。当时计划去很多地方，想了很多个目的地，只是想最后 final 结束的时候再确定一个。但是因为得了我也没有太敢找她，而且她也正好没有来找我，所以…

Yes, both of us got Covid-19. At that time, we planned to go to many places and thought of many destinations, just to pick one after the final week. Then I got Covid-19 and I didn't dare to contact her, and she also happened never to contact me, so...

[00:18:42.15] Yiwen: 这件事情就这么鸽掉了？

The whole plan was just canceled.

[00:18:43.04] 71: 对，就鸽掉了。我后来才知道，她也得了，她也，对。

Yes, just canceled. It was a long time before I heard that she also got Covid-19 at that time.

[00:18:47.01] Yiwen: 而且她也没有告诉你她得了这件事情？

And she didn't tell you?

[00:18:49.01] 71: 对，她没有告诉我，是我自己知道，因为我也没有告诉她，因为我跟他就没有接触嘛。她不是我的密接，我就没有必要跟她说。

Yes, she never told me. I heard it from someone else. And I never told her about my getting Covid-19 because I didn't meet her during that time. She was not a close contact of me and there was no need to tell her.

[00:18:57.16] Yiwen: 在得过新冠这件事情之后，感染过一次之后，你在对待疫情的态度上面会有一些改变吗？

After getting Covid-19, has your attitude to this virus changed?

[00:19:05.05] 71: 我觉得这个是看前后期吧。刚刚得，是在我得中和得后和得后很久之后都有变化。得中的时候，我当时是想等我痊愈，如果我有机会痊愈，我当时觉得可能还没机会痊愈来着。（笑）对，我当时是觉得如果我有机会痊愈，我再也不再去高风险的地方，我可能又会变成我刚来美国的时候那种非常谨慎的态度。对。在我得后的，不，痊愈之后，我当时就想，痊愈了，那，因为当时自我隔离了，我觉得快一个月了，我当时也确实觉得有点闷了。我是觉得我可以出去透透气。我是这样觉得。但是我也不会去太危险的地方。主要是我还知道一个信息，如果你得过，你当时的抗体浓度会比较高。

I think this also changed with different periods. When I first got it, or during my illness and after I was cured, and long after I was cured, there were changes. When I was sick, I was thinking that if I had a chance to recover, I even thought about the possibility that I could never recover. (Laughs) I was thinking that if I had a chance to get cured, I would never go back to a high-risk place again, and I would probably become the very cautious person I was when I first came to the U.S. Then after I got, I mean, recovered, I was like, because of the long self-quarantine, I did feel a bit bored at the time, and I thought I should go out and breathe some fresh air. But I wouldn't go anywhere dangerous. And I heard that if you just recovered, the antibody concentration in your blood would be higher.

[00:19:57.20] Yiwen: 就是短期内你不容易…

It means in a short term, you would not…

[00:19:59.06] 71: 对对对。你的风险是比没得过的人应该是低很多对。就是有这种双重保障吧，所以我当时还选择出去透透气。而且正好我当时，那个得过的那个同学，跟我一起计划出游的同学，她也痊愈了，所以基本上我们两个一起在附近逛了一下，但是也没有，也不太敢去太远的地方。在得过很久之后，第三个阶段基本上已经忘了自己得过对事情。对，基本上又恢复，想要，觉得去哪里都可以的这种情况。

Yes. Your risk would be much lower than other people's. That's why I chose to go out and get some fresh air at that time. And coincidentally, the friend who also got Covid, the one I was planning a trip with, also recovered. And we had a very short trip near New York together for we still didn't dare to go too far away. Then, after recovering for a long time, it comes to the third stage. I almost forget I once got Covid-19 and it goes back to the situation that I feel I can go anywhere I want.

[00:20:33.15] Yiwen: ，所以就开始计划下一次的长途的旅行？

And you are planning another long trip?

[00:20:36.20] 71: 对对对，又变成这种情况了。

Yes, it's turning into this status again.

[00:20:38.10] Yiwen: 你有告诉你的家人，你感染这件事情吗？

Have you ever told your parents that you got Covid-19?

[00:20:41.14] 71: 没有。得的时候，我觉得告诉他们没有太大的用处，只会让他们担心，甚至他们会觉得我出国这个决定，可能会直接上升到这种，否定你出国这种决定。对。我痊愈之后，我觉得就更没有必要说了，因为你已经好了，没有什么事情，我觉得就更没有必要再把这件事情说出来。对。

Never. When I was sick, I felt it could not help in any sense by telling them but only making them worry. They may even question my decision of coming to the U.S. After I recovered, there was even less need to tell them because you have already recovered.

[00:21:07.22] Yiwen: 所以你的家人至今都不知道你曾经短暂得阳性过？

So your parents still don't know that you once tested positive?

[00:21:11.24] 71: 至今都不知道，但是我可能有时候会差点说漏嘴。我当时感冒的时候，我会问他们我需要吃什么药缓解我的症状，他们就会语气比较僵硬，他们觉得我可能应该是得了新冠，非常礼貌地跟我说你要不要去测一下，（笑）我就说我已经约上了。我约上的时候他就会一直问我什么时候去测，我告诉他们的时候之后又说结果什么时候出来。每次打电话都会非常地关心我最终的结果。如我最后告诉

他们是阴性的时候,他会有一种很奇怪感觉,就算我告诉他是阴性,他还是不相信。

They don't know so far, but I may have almost let it slip sometimes. When I thought it was just the flu, I once asked them what medicine to take, and they were nervous. They thought it might be Covid-19 and asked me to get tested in a very cautious manner, (laughs) and I told them I already made an appointment. Then they kept asking me when the appointment would be and when the result would come out. Every time I called them, they would ask about the test result. I lied to them and said it was negative, but I was not sure whether they believed me.

[00:21:55.18] Yiwen: 他们有让你再去测一次吗?

Did they ask you to go for another test?

[00:21:58.23] 71: 他甚至觉得我要么是没去测,要么就是测出来结果是不对的,要么就是告诉他们谎话。或者种种原因,就是我感觉我陷入一种,我不管说什么,他们就会觉得你只要感冒了,你可能,对。他说,甚至他觉得就算你是阴性,你现在感冒了,你的抵抗力可能也比较差。所以你还是需要警惕。

They even felt like I might never go for the test, or the result was wrong, or I lied to them. I felt like I went into a kind of situation where they didn't care what I said. As long as I had those symptoms, it should be Covid. And they even believed that even my test result was really negative, I was still in extreme danger because the flu lowered my immunity.

[00:22:20.22] Yiwen: 其实我跟你讲，我这学期发烧了好几次，就很低很低的低烧。正好有一天跟我妈在视频的时候，我觉得我不太舒服，好像有点发烧，我自己有体温计，我就跟我妈说我可能有点发烧，我妈说你赶快测一下，就测了，确实是在发烧。我妈就非常非常恐慌。当时我家有自测盒，我说你别担心，我现在测一下，我这一期已经不是第一次发烧了，我就是玩累了，我就会发烧，我说你别担心，我去做一个自测。我就当着我妈的面把整个自测流程做完，她一直跟我视频着，等它15分钟出结果，一直到出结果把展示给我妈看。我当时其实就在想，万一我这是个阳性。我妈见证了整个全程，我被阳对全过程，我都没办法骗她了。你知道吗？我就特别后悔我跟我妈说，我现在觉得有点发烧。（71: 对。）就是你真的不能告诉他们你有任何的那种…

In fact, I got a fever many times this semester, a very low fever. And one day I was having face timing with my mom, and I felt not so good, like a fever. I had a thermometer at home. I told my mom I might have a fever and she asked me to check my temperature and it turned out to be a fever. My mom was in a panic. I told her not to worry and that I had a self-test kit at home, and I could do a test and show her I was just too tired and got a fever. So I did the self-test with Facetime on and my mom waited 15 minutes to see the result. I was thinking that if the result was positive, then my mom would have witnessed the whole process of my testing positive, and there would be no way for me to hide it from her. And I was so regret telling her I might have a fever at first. (71: I feel you!) It's like you can never tell them that you have…

[00:23:13.12] 71: 发烧的症状。这种对我觉得也不只是你的家里人，甚至你身边的同学，你都要慎用发烧这个字眼。

Any symptom like fever. And I think you have to be cautious about using the word 'fever' not just with your family, but even with your friends around you.

[00:23:23.04] Yiwen: 在我被你告知你得新冠这件事情之后，我跟我妈聊天时候说漏嘴了。

And after I was told you got Covid-19, I accidentally let my mom know.

[00:23:30.27] 71: 你说我有，你有一个朋友得新冠了？

You told her that one of your friends got Covid-19?

[00:23:33.15] Yiwen: 对。（笑）我一开始以为不会有什么大事的嘛，（71: 哦。）但是就是我妈说你快去做个核酸检测啊。你别那个了。我做了核酸检测她也不相信。（71: 笑）一定要把那个截图，就是真的把邮件的 PDF 吧好像，还是网页的截图，发给她。她其实不懂英语，但是她可以用翻译软件看嘛。她看到 negative 她才放心。然后我就觉得如果我真的得了的话，我好像可能没有办法瞒得住他们。

Yes. (Laugh.) At first, I thought it would be fine. (71: Em.) But my mom asked me to do a test as soon as possible just in case. And after I tested negative, she didn't believe in me. (71: Laugh.) She asked me to share the screenshot of the email or the pdf document of the result with her. She could not read English, but she could use translation software. She wasn't relieved until she saw the word 'negative'. Then then I felt if I really got Covid-19, there may not really be a way to hide the truth from them.

[00:24:10.15] (Music)

Vol-4 Zoey

一年网课一年线下，她如何看待两者的优劣?

One year online and one year offline, how does this girl see these two modes?

Zoey: Zoey graduated from a college in Shanghai as an undergraduate and the University of Michigan, Ann Arbor as a graduate student. After a year of online, she finally came to the United States and took the second half of classes of her master's program onsite. In her first year of the master's program, she often needed to stay up very late at night to take classes due to the time difference. For this reason, she even moved to live in the countryside for some days. At the time of this interview, Zoey had graduated and returned to Shanghai to work.

[00:00:00.00] (Music)

[00:00:04.26] VoiceOver: 欢迎来到 The Two Years Stolen，我是 Yiwen。

Welcome to The Two Years Stolen, I'm Yiwen.

[00:00:15.15] VoiceOver: 这一期的受访者是我的高中同学 Zoey。Zoey 本科毕业于上海的一所高校，研究生则毕业于密歇根大学安娜堡分校。在接受这段采访的时候，Zoey 已经毕业回到上海工作。

The interviewee of this episode is Zoey, a high school friend of mine. Zoey graduated from a college in Shanghai as an undergraduate and the University of Michigan, Ann Arbor as a graduate student. At the time of this interview, Zoey had graduated and returned to Shanghai to work.

[00:00:27.27] (Music)

[00:00:30.24] VoiceOver: Zoey 从大三开始准备留学的相关事宜，到疫情爆发的时候，她已经基本上完成了所有的申请过程。

Zoey began preparing for studying abroad in her junior year, and by the time the pandemic broke out, she had almost completed all of the application processes.

[00:00:39.06] Yiwen: 你是大概什么时候开始想要出国留学的？

When did you begin to think about studying abroad?

[00:00:42.25] Zoey: 我是在本科大三的时候开始有这个想法，并且开始准备一些语言考试。

My junior year. And I began to prepare for the language tests since then.

[00:00:50.05] Yiwen: 为什么想要出国留学？

Why do you want to study abroad?

[00:00:51.14] Zoey: 因为就是觉得出国留学算是一种学历，一方面是为了学历提升，拿一个硕士学位，另一个就是我在本科阶段有过一段在英国的交换的经历，让我觉得自己还蛮想去国外完整地读一个学位。这样差不多两个主要的原因。我当时其实英国和美国有一起申请，英国也有申请，大概三四所。美国是申请得比较多，申了七八所，大概主要是申美国。英国当时是作为一个保底的选择。想去美国是因为美国学制比较长嘛，一般都是两年或者一年。

On the one hand, it's some kind of improvement of my educational background, I wanted to get a master's degree. The other reason is that I had an exchange experience in the UK in college, which made me feel that I quite wanted to study abroad for longer. These were the two main reasons. At that time, I actually applied to schools in both the U.K. and the

U.S., three or four in the U.K., and seven or eight in the U.S. The U.K. schools were guaranteed choice. I wanted to go to the U.S. because the length of schooling in the U.S. is longer, usually two years or one year and a half.

[00:01:33.21] Yiwen: 那你还记得 2020 年，当时疫情刚刚爆发的时候，你在哪？你在做些什么？

Do you still remember where you were and what you were doing when the pandemic broke out in 2020?

[00:01:39.01] Zoey: 我记得疫情刚刚爆发，差不多是当年（2019 年）11 月还是 12 月的时候，当时我是，正好是寒假，就没有课了，因为我们学校，本科学校是三学期制，当时正好是假期，我就回江苏的老家了。疫情爆发的时候正好是在家里。

I think the pandemic began in November or December of 2019.[3] It was winter break for me. My school runs on a trimester system, and it happened to be our winter break. I have been back to my hometown in Jiangsu and I was there when the pandemic broke out.

[00:02:01.00] Yiwen: 当时你的申请进入到一个什么阶段？

To what stage did your application reach at that time?

[00:02:03.06] Zoey: 我当时的申请差不多都已经，呃，应该是都已经交了申请了，差不多交了。对，后面没有交的，因为都是，语言，当时也有了，雅思也有了，所以一些网上操作的提交，所以对我申请这一步其实影响没有那么大。

---

[3] The pandemic began in December 2019, but at that time most people didn't pay much attention to it because the official medias in China called it a rumor.

I have submitted almost all the applications. Even for the applications that I haven't submitted yet, I already have language scores, like IELTS, and the only thing I needed to do is to fill out the application form online. So, pandemic didn't affect the process of my application.

[00:02:24.25] Yiwen: 你在 20 年的时候，疫情刚刚爆发的时候，你有过一个对于疫情大概什么时候可以结束这件事情的预期吗？

Did you have an expectation of when the pandemic would be over at that time?

[00:02:33.10] Zoey: 我当时以为过了年就会好的，但是没有。因为当时过年的时候我记得是我们大四是吧，就大四那年，我当时以为过了年开学了它就正常了，没想到一直到我，到我毕业它都没有好。

I thought everything would be fine after Spring Festival. But as you can see, it didn't. I was in my junior year. I thought the pandemic would end before the beginning of my last trimester in college. I never expect it would last till now after I graduated from graduate school.

[00:02:52.28] Yiwen: 你大四的下学期是在家上网课的吗？还是有机会回到学校？

You were taking online classes at home in your last trimester? Or have you had a chance to go back to campus?

[00:02:58.09] Zoey: 我当时是没有课了，基本上就在家里，然后也，回学校是 6 月份去参加的毕业典礼。对，其实没有，我们没有毕业典礼，相当于一个去拍个照片，就回学校回了 3 天收拾东西，主要是收拾东西。

I had no classes in that trimester and I almost stayed at home the whole trimester. And I went back to campus in June to attend the graduation ceremony. In fact, we didn't have a graduation ceremony. We only went back and took some photos and only stayed there for 3 days, mainly for packaging my luggage.

[00:03:15.01] VoiceOver: Zoey 介绍称，自己的学校当时提供了 defer 的选项，但她依旧选择了先上一年网课。

Zoey told me that though the University of Michigan, Ann Arbor did provide the choice of deferral, she took online classes for the first year.

[00:03:21.23] Zoey: 当时是有给我们 defer 的，就是晚一年入学的一个选择。但是我们有大概 1/3 的人是选择晚一年入学。我们也有 6 个中国学生，我们是选择的上，读网课。上网课。

They provided the choice of deferral, which means we could register one year later. About one-third of the students deferred, while 6 Chinese students, including me, were taking online classes.

[00:03:40.02] Yiwen: 你当时为什么选择上网课？

Why did you make that choice?

[00:03:41.26] Zoey: 因为当时觉得如果 defer 也，疫情也待在家里也挺无聊的，还不如就上网课。而且我本身是两年嘛，想着一年上网课，还有一年至少还可以出去。

I felt it might be boring to stay at home for a whole year. And my program was a two-year program. Even if I had online classes for one year, I could at least go offline for another year.

[00:03:56.16] Yiwen: 你上网课当时会有遇到一些时差的问题，需要在国内的夜间上课吗？

Did you meet any problem with the time difference, like having to attending classes at midnight?

[00:04:04.29] Zoey: 需要的。我当时很多课都是晚上 9 点钟开始，上到第二天凌晨 3、4 点这样。

Yes. Many classes began from 9 p.m. and would last till 3 or 4 a.m. next day.

[00:04:12.04] Yiwen: 你是怎么来调整作息的？

What did you do to get adjusted?

[00:04:16.18] Zoey: 硬调整。当时因为我在家里的话，比较影响我爸妈的生活，后来我一开始是先去我爷爷奶奶家住，后来我就自己一个人住。一个人这样作息就不会影响别人，吃饭的话，外卖或者是点熟食。

I just forced myself to adapt. And if I stayed at home and stayed up late every day, I may influence my parents' life. So I moved to live with my grandparents at first. Then, I moved out to live alone to reduce the influence on others. And during the days I lived alone, I ordered delivery everyday.

[00:04:37.24] Yiwen: 你觉得网课的体验和你第二年线下上课的体验相比，各自的优势和缺陷在哪？

What do you think are the strengths and weaknesses of the online class experience compared to your second-year offline class experience?

[00:04:44.28] Zoey: 网课？其实，网课的优势就在于我没有那么重的语言上或者是各方面的压力，因为毕竟是一个线上的课程，没有那种环境给我的压力。所以对我来说，当时第一年网课纯粹就是学业、作业、考试之类的一些困难，不用去融入环境，或者去跟同学交流，或跟舍友相处这种情况。这是我可能觉得它唯一的好处，但它的…而且我自己是比较幸运，我在网课那年，我遇到一个比较好的一个教授，他当时是考虑到我们凌晨5点钟上课，他给，后来他是给我们调了课程时间。当时我他班上是两个中国学生，我还有另外一个人，我们两个是每周五的上午上课，相当于他用晚上的时间来给我们上课。后来因为每周我们三个人交流时间比较长，后来我们就成了比较好的朋友。我后来刚去美国的时候，线下上课的第一年，因为有提前认识这样一个比较好的老师，所以给了我们很多的帮助，包括我后面回国，当时考虑申请别的项目，都受了很多帮助。所以我可能觉得线上上课带给我比较好的两个地方。但是坏处就是没有上学的体验感，没有同学，没有任何学校的好玩的活动，还蛮可惜的。

Online classes? Actually, the advantage of online classes was that I didn't have the pressure of language, because after all, it was online, and I didn't have the pressure adapting to a different language environment. So, for me, the first year of online classes was purely about academics, assignments, exams, without having to integrate into the environment or communicate with my classmates or get along with roommates. That's the only advantage, but it's...And I was lucky to have a very nice professor in the year of online classes. He thought it would be too tiring for us to attend classes at 5 a.m., and he offered to give us classes at a different time. There were two Chinese students in that class, me and another person. So the professor rescheduled the class for us two every Friday morning which was equivalent to him using the evening hours to give us classes separately. Because the three of us spent more time together each week, we became good friends. When I first went to the U.S., during my first year of offline classes, I got to know such a good teacher in advance, so he gave us a lot of help, including when I made the decision to return to China, and when I was considering applying to other programs, he helped a lot. So I think the online classes brought me two good things. But the drawback is that there are no sense of school experience, no classmates, and no fun school activities, which is quite a pity.

[00:06:25.02] Yiwen: 这个教授他是单独给你们两个人调了时间，（Zoey：对。）其他的同学，他会先上一遍，再给你们两个上。

So the professor rescheduled the class for only two of you? (Zoey: Yes.) He first gave classes to all other students, then two of you again separately?

[00:06:32.29] Zoey: 再给我们上一遍。对，因为那门课上就两个中国学生，所以他是给其他大概十来个人上一遍，星期五再给我们两个单独上一遍。

He gave us the lessons again. Because there were only two Chinese students in that class, he had to give the lessons to the other ten students, and then separately for us on Friday.

[00:06:42.12] Yiwen: 那这个其实还蛮辛苦的，相当于是他又增加了，比如两个小时（Zoey：对。）或者3个小时左右的工作。

That would be tiring. (Zoey: Yes.) Like adding two to three hours a week to his workload.

[00:06:49.12] Zoey: 对,是这样。所以我们每周我们小的聊天特别多,后来大家关系就变得比较好。

Yes. And this means we can have some more small talks every week, which brought us closer together.

[00:06:57.27] Yiwen: 你现在再回想一下,你 20 年的时候决定上网课的决定,你觉得这是你在当时做出的最正确的决定吗?

So, do you think it is the best choice you could made in 2020?

[00:07:06.01] Zoey: 如果是现在的我不会上网课,但是对于当时的我来说,我觉得网课也没什么不好的。因为现在我可能觉得我会用那一年的时间去做几份,做几份实习,或者考两个证之类的。但是当时的我其实没有很强的为了以后就业做打算的概念,因为我没有,一开始没有就业的打算。我打算讲、继续读书。所以如果让当时的我去选择 Defer 一年,我可能一年就在家里,或者去找一份不一定特别适合未来找工作的实习,所以我觉得可能差别也不大,所以还好吧。

If it was now, I wouldn't have taken online classes, but for me at that time, I don't think there was anything wrong with online classes. Because now I may think I will use that year to do a few internships or obtain two certificates or something like that. But at that time, I actually did not have a very strong concept of making plans for future employment, because I did not, at first, have any intention of employment. I planned to stay in school and keep studying. So if I chose to defer for a year, I might stay at home for a year but do nothing, or find an internship that is not suitable for future job hunting. So, if I had another chance, I might make a same choice.

[00:07:55.01] Yiwen: 之前说你之前的计划是继续读书，是再读一个硕士还是读 PhD？（Zoey：PhD。）你现在还想读 PhD 吗？

You said you planned to stay in school and keep studying, does that mean pursuing another master's degree or Ph.D. degree? (Zoey: Ph.D.) Do you still want to pursue a Ph.D. degree?

[00:08:07.23] Zoey: 现在还没想好，因为我当时，我是去年没有，我是没有参加秋招。因为我当时秋招的时候在准备 PhD 的申请。在我找老师给我写推荐信的时候跟他聊了一下，他当时，他是建议我一定要工作两年再决定要不要读 PhD。我觉得挺有道理的，反正工作两年再读也不是不可以。后来我就去春招，就开始找工作。

Haven't decided yet. Last year, I missed the autumn recruitment. I was preparing for the application for Ph.D. during the autumn recruitment period. But I had a talk with my professor when I asked for a recommendation letter from him. He suggested that I work for two years before deciding whether I really want a PhD degree. I thought it also made sense. So I participated in the spring recruitment and found a job.

[00:08:36.26] Yiwen: 你后来申请了吗？

So, did you apply at last?

[00:08:38.29] Zoey: 后来没有申请，（笑）就是找推荐信那一步，跟他聊了一下，觉得他说的好有道理，我就没有再申请。因为我觉得很奇怪，我其实 PhD，我是觉得当所有人觉得我该读的时候，我就会去申请，包括我爸我妈觉得我该读，我就

去申请。但是一旦有一个人觉得你可以再想想，我立马就会说那我就再想想。其实我后来发现，我其实内心没有那么坚定地想要。

No. (Laugh.) I was persuaded by him and gave up all the applications. I think I'm a very indecisive person that when everyone, including my parents insisted that I should study for a PhD degree, I would apply for it. But once there is someone suggested me rethinking, I would give up without any hesitate. And I realized afterward, I didn't want it that badly.

[00:09:07.05] VoiceOver: 因为我们在差不多的时间赴美，又在临近的时期从美国回到中国。所以 Zoey 和我分享了我们赴美以及回国的一些经历，以及我们在美期间身边的人对于新冠疫情的态度。

Since Zoey and I departure to the U.S. and came back to China both at approximately the same time, we shared some related experiences, and the attitudes of the people around us to the Covid-19 when we were in the U.S.

[00:09:22.04] Zoey: 我是在 21 年的 7 月，呃，8 月份去的美国。

I went to the U.S. in July, no, August 2021.

[00:09:29.13] Yiwen: 之前办签证的时候，因为我印象当中大使馆是到 5 月份才开的。

Did the visa application go smoothly? Because I have the impression that the embassy did not open until May.

[00:09:35.09] Zoey: 是。我当时是抢到了上海的一个签证吧。好像当时在上海办的签证，抢到之后，我运气比较好，没有被取消，所以就签证还行，没有很困难。

Yes. I was able to get a visa appointment in Shanghai, I think. I was lucky enough not to have my appointment cancelled, so it was fine and not very difficult.

[00:09:51.22] Yiwen: 在大使馆开放之前，你有考虑过去一些其他的国家办理签证这样子的过程吗？因为我记得我当时还约了同学，如果它到 5 月份还不开，我们就会一起去新加坡，在新加坡办好了签证，直接从新加坡飞美国。这样的。

Before the embassy opened, did you consider going to a third country to get a visa as a plan B? Because I remember, I planned to go to Singapore together with a friend to get a visa there and fly directly to the U.S. It was our plan.

[00:10:11.05] Zoey: 没有考虑过。因为当时其实我就想着如果再在家里读一年，我就升我们学校的二专，我再读一个专业，用一年，这样子也一样可以出去，所以没有那么着急。因为我们学校比较鼓励读二专，我其实 80% 的同学都会修第二个硕士学位，所以没有那么急着想，如果万一办不了，就第二年再去就好了。

I didn't consider about it. I was thinking that if I had to stay at home for another year, I could apply for a second master's program in our school. In this way, I could still study offline in the U.S. for at least one year. Our school really encourages students to pursue a second master's degree and 80% of my classmates are pursuing their second master's degree. Considering this, I was not that worried. If I could not get a visa, I would go to the U.S. the next year.

[00:10:38.04] Yiwen: 所以其实你原本是觉得在家上两年网课也是可以接受的？

So you felt it was acceptable to take online classes at home for two years?

[00:10:42.11] Zoey: 嗯，那我可以再读一个二专，再出去，申一个二专，再出去也可以。我，因为我只我当时想觉得不可能持续3年，但是没想到他确实是持续了3年。

Yes. I could apply for a second master's program and go to the U.S. then. And I thought the pandemic would not last for three years, but it did last for three years.

[00:10:54.20] Yiwen: 你到美国之后，你对自己在新冠的防护上面，你有做一些比较特别的事情吗？

Did you do any special preparation on the protection when you departure to the U.S.?

[00:11:03.12] Zoey: 没有，我其实决定去美国的时候起，我自己对于这件事情就比较随遇而安。戴口罩对我就是我唯一做的事情。什么眼罩，防护服，什么巴拉巴拉，其他所有东西我都没有准备。我就觉得该戴口罩的时候戴口罩，我该做的做了，其他就无所谓。

No. From the moment I decided to go, I didn't care too much. Wearing masks was the only thing I did. I didn't prepare anything else like Protective Goggles, Protective clothing, or any other things. I thought if I could wear masks whenever it was needed, the was out of my control.

[00:11:24.26] Yiwen: 你周围有朋友感染过？

Do you have any friend who got Covid-19?

[00:11:28.06] Zoey: 有，我室友当时就感染了。我住的是2B2B，我室友就感染了。

Yes, my roommate once got. I lived in a 2B2B, and my roommate was test positive someday.

[00:11:34.12] Yiwen: 2B2B 的话，其实你们应该是要共用厨房和客厅？

2B2B means you had to share the kitchen and the living room with her?

[00:11:37.21] Zoey: 对，但是她，我没有被感染，或者我被感染过，但是我自己不知道。所以我，所有我在美国做的检测，我都是阴性，但我觉得我可能会感染过，毕竟中招的人太多了。

Yes. But I was not infected. Or I was once infected, but I didn't know. All the tests I did in the U.S. turned out to be negative. But maybe I have gotten Covid some time, after all, too many people have gotten.

[00:11:53.10] Yiwen: 你室友感染的时候，你们有做一些特殊的这种措施来保证你们俩没有接触吗？还是就是…

Did you take any special measures to ensure no exposure to her when your roommate got Covid? Or you just…

[00:12:02.19] Zoey: 感染的时候我们就错开吃饭，她去食堂，她去客厅、厨房吃饭的时候我就在房间里，我吃饭的时候他就在房间。

We had meals at different times. When she went to the living room and the kitchen for food, I would stay in my bedroom. And when I went out for meals, she would stay in her room.

[00:12:13.21] Yiwen: 有那段时间会有使劲地在厨房，比如消毒，或者这些她用完之后，还有你进去之前。

Did you sanitize more in the kitchen and living room, especially after she used it and before you got into it?

[00:12:20.05] Zoey: 好像也没有。（笑）因为我当时也比较佛系，她自己比我更在意一点，她人还蛮好的，她怕传染给我，其实我觉得还好。

I don't think so. (Laugh.) I didn't care too much. And it seems that she cared more about it. She is nice and she was afraid to infect me. But I was ok with it.

[00:12:32.06] Yiwen: 我当时住的是一个 3B1B。圣诞节的前期，我的一个好朋友感染了，其实我和那个好朋友应该很久没有见了，但就在我那个朋友在被测出阳性的那一天，我跟那个朋友约饭，但是最后也没有约得成。因为我当时是有一些事情，所以我去晚了。我那个朋友她自己已经吃得快要吃完了，我们只是打了个招呼。所以我们俩可能也不能算是非常严格意义上的密接，因为我们俩就是戴着口罩讲了两句话而已。但是这个事情之后，我告诉了我的室友，我的其中一个室友，她就非常的紧张。她是一个印度人，可能她自己家人在 20 年的时候，可能像她的哥哥还有什么家人可能都感染过，而且他们当时感染的应该是 Delta，比较严重的一种吧。而且她也见，因为她 20 年的时候也在印度，她见证了印度整个状况比较严重的时期，所以她非常的恐惧，她当时就被吓得要死。虽然我知道你跟你的朋友其实没有太多的接触，但是万一呢？你一定要去给我做检测，而且因为我们是 3B1B，我们得共用卫生间这些。她要求我用完卫生间之后一定要用所有消毒剂喷好各种。但是后来很快我测了两次，而且她让我一定要测两次，她说一次可能会不准，或者是有潜伏期，所以她让我测两次。我做。我在家里进行了一个 self-quarantine，大概做

了两天还是三天。然后我没有事情之后，她就开始跟我一起玩了。但我好像，他们都说这些外国人可能不在乎或者什么，但是我身边遇到过的最 care 这件事情的其实是一个印度人。对。

I was living in a 3B1B, and right before Christmas last year, one of my friends got Covid. I hadn't seen her for a long time, but it was the day she tested positive, I initially planned to have lunch with her, though it didn't work out. I was late because of some urgent matter. She had almost finished the meal when I arrived, and we only said hello to each other. So, the two of us might not be considered as close contact, because we both wore masks and spoke only a few words. But after she tested positive, I told my roommates. One of them got very nervous. She's an Indian, and some of her family members, like her brother once got Covid in 2020. And it should be Delta, a more serious kind of virus. And she also saw, because she was in India in 2020, she witnessed the whole situation in India in a more serious period. So, she was very scared. She was like although I know you didn't really have much contact with your friend, what if the virus is so strong? You must go and get tested. And we were living in a 3B1B, which means we had to share bathrooms. She asked me to make sure to sanitize the bathroom thoroughly every time after using it. And I was asked to test twice because she believed only testing once might be inaccurate or there might be an incubation period. I did, I also did a self-quarantine at home for about two or three days. And then after seeing the two test results, she finally got relieved and began to hang out with me again. People always say that only the Chinese care about this virus, but the one I've met that cares the most is actually an Indian.

[00:14:14.17] Zoey: 我其实身边遇到过的最 care 疫情的是我老师。因为他是 49 年出生的，他年纪也，他是属于他自己，非常非常在意疫情。我每次跟他在外面一起喝咖啡或者吃饭，他都一定要坐在室外，会戴好口罩，只要是离开座位就会戴好口罩，像包括上课的时候都会一直紧紧戴着那种，我忘记叫啥了，KN（Yiwen: N95 吗？）对，差不多是那种。我觉得他是我遇到最在意的这个事情的美国人。

The person I know who is most concerned about this virus is my teacher. He was born in 1949 and he is quite old. So, he cares about the virus so much. Every time we had coffee, or dinner outside, he would request to sit outdoors and wear a mask. I mean, as long as he left the table, he would wear a mask. And of course, in class, he would always wear the mask, KN? I cannot remember the name. (Yiwen: N95.) Yes, that kind of mask. He is the American who cares about the virus the most I've ever met.

[00:14:49.18] Yiwen: 你是什么时候回到上海的？

And when did you come back to Shanghai?

[00:14:51.10] Zoey: 我是今年 6 月底。我买了直飞的机票，所以我当时是直接从底特律飞上海。飞到上海之后，当时的隔离政策是 3+4。我在上海隔离 3 天，在我江苏的老家隔离 4 天。是这样的。

Late this June. It was a non-stop flight, from Detroit to Shanghai. And the quarantine policy was 3+4 at that time. I had a 3-day quarantine in Shanghai, then a 4-day one in my hometown in Jiangsu. That's my experience.

[00:15:12.28] Yiwen: 是酒店隔离还是居家？

In a hotel or at home?

[00:15:14.16] Zoey: 都是酒店隔离。回，3 天上海的酒店，4 天江苏的酒店，然后再居家隔离 3 天。3 +4+3 这样。

Both were in hotels. 3 days in a hotel in Shanghai, and 4 days in a hotel in Jiangsu. Then I had to take a 3-day self-quarantine at home. It should be 3+4+3.

[00:15:24.14] Yiwen: 我后来回来的时候好像当时是直接的 7+3。当然我还经过了香港的过程。

When I came back, it was directly 7+3. But I flew to Hong Kong first.

[00:15:30.29] Zoey: 我没有经过香港，我是直接到上海，因为当时只允许直飞，没有办法。

I didn't go to Hong Kong, but directly to Shanghai. Only non-stop flights were allowed at that time and I had no choice.

[00:15:37.18] Yiwen: 我是很早就买了直飞的机票，当时是从洛杉矶直飞，好像是天津，应该是北京的，它是天津入境，所以应该是洛杉矶直飞天津。结果在我开始准备收拾行李去洛杉矶住一个月的时候，我收到了通知，它告诉我说你的航拍被熔断了。

I bought a non-stop flight very early. And it was from Los Angeles to Tianjin. It should be Beijing but would first stop in Tianjin. [4] However, when I was packing my luggage

---

[4] It was a policy in China to protect Beijing as the capital. All the international flights to Beijing would first stop in another city in China and all the passengers could get to Beijing after the quarantine in a hotel.

and planned to fly to Los Angeles and live there for a month, [5] I was noticed that my flight was cancelled. [6]

[00:16:00.10] Zoey: 哦？是的，太恶心了。当时底特律一个礼拜好像只有两趟航班可以飞，283 和 287，太恐怖了，而且机票好贵。

Oh? That's annoying. And I remember there were only two flights from Detroit to Shanghai every week, the flight number was 283 and 287. And it was far from enough. And the tickets were so expensive.

[00:16:13.06] Yiwen: 我当时它一下子熔断了 4 班。所以后来我就想，我就说，那个时候已经可以从香港转了嘛。很多人都走叫"猪肝红计划"，我就开始搜各种资料怎么来猪肝红。后来是 9 月初的时候回来的。

Yes. And I remember I met a huge cancellation of 4 flight. So I finally decided to transfer in Hong Kong. at that time, people were allowed not to take a non-stop flight and many people transferred in Hong Kong. They call this routine "Pork Liver Red Plan"[7] , and you could find a lot of tips. And I finally got home in September.

[00:16:31.11] Zoey: 那还好，还算顺利，你回来了。

That's great. At least you come back successfully.

[00:16:35.27] (Music)

---

[5] There was a time in China when the policy required that you could not leave the place of departure for a week or so before the exact departure day. This meant that I had to be in Los Angeles sometime earlier.

[6] There was a policy that if the amount of positive cases in one international flight reached a certain number, the Chinese government would cancel the next 2 or 4 flights with the same flight number as a penalty to the airline.

[7] People who take this routine would get a red QR Code on their way home, and the color was close to pork liver.

Vol-5 Lily

放弃出国回国到家乡当公务员，她如何看待当初的这一决定？

Giving up the chance to study abroad but working as a civil servant, how does she see this choice?

Lily: Lily graduated from Nanjing University in 2020. She initially planned to go to Hong Kong or Singapore for a master's degree and did receive some offers. However, the uncertainty of the pandemic made her reject all the offers and went back to her hometown. She is now working as a civil servant in the local government. She has given up the idea of studying abroad but is thinking about attending a part-time master's program in China.

[00:00:00.00] (Music)

[00:00:04.26] VoiceOver: 欢迎来到 The Two Years Stolen，我是 Yiwen。

Welcome to The Two Years Stolen, I'm Yiwen.

[00:00:15.15] VoiceOver: 这一期的受访者是我的高中同学 Lily。从南京大学毕业后，因为疫情的影响和家人的坚持，她放弃了前往新加坡留学的机会，而选择回到家乡做一名公务员。

The interviewee of this episode is my high school classmate, Lily. After graduating from Nanjing University in 2020, she gave up the chance to study in Singapore due to the pandemic and her parents' suggestions and went back to her hometown, working as a civil servant in the local government.

[00:00:29.16] (Music)

[00:00:32.13] VoiceOver: 在采访中，Lily 与我分享了她从计划留学到最终放弃留学计划回到家乡的全部过程。

In the interview, Lily shared the whole process from her planning to study abroad to finally rejecting the offer and going back to her hometown.

[00:00:40.12] Lily: 具体应该还是在大三下学期的时候开始的。我大二的时候从学校的交换项目网站上看到了一个，浏览了一下，参加了一个交换项目。大二暑假的时候是去加拿大的 UBC，就是英属哥伦比亚大学进行了一个短期的交换。这一段是相当于一段类似于开阔眼界的那种经历。大概知道了一下，大概国外的大学是什么样子的一个上课的方式。到大三下学期的时候，那个时候我在实习。因为专业的缘故，我是南京大学新闻传播学院的，我们学院是江苏广播电视总台跟南京大学部校共建的这样的一个学院。所以我那个时候是在江苏电视台进行一个实习。实习完了之后就开始思考我，我是继续读硕士还是找工作还是考研。然后思考了一下，不是很想考研，我说那就选择出国。我主要是申请的香港和新加坡的学校，因为这样，一个是时间也比较短，基本上是一年制的。第二个是离家近。离家近不会有太多的时差什么，跟家里联系也比较方便一点。当时基本上就是香港的前面 5 所，还有新加坡的 2 所都申请了。大概在大四上半学期的时候，应该是拿到了港中文和香港科技大学的 offer，当面后面的什么城市大学的也有，反正除了港大吧。（笑）但是那个时候大概是，好像是，我不太确定。那个时候你知道香港在暴动，有段时间。港中文那个时候他们在搞独立，好像是大家就都不太放心去香港。也有很多拿到了港校 offer 的同学都在观望，不确定要不要去，那个时候。

I began to prepare in the second semester of my junior year. When I was a sophomore, I saw browsed through my school's exchange program website and joined an exchange program. During the summer of my sophomore year, I went to UBC, aka the University of British Columbia in Canada, for a short-term exchange program. This was more like an eye-opening experience. I got to know about the way of teaching in universities abroad. In the second semester of my junior year, I was doing an internship at that time. Because of my major, I am from the School of Journalism and Communication of Nanjing University, which is a school established jointly by Jiangsu Radio and Television and Nanjing University. So, I was doing an internship at Jiangsu TV Station at that time. After the internship, I started to think about whether I should study abroad or find a job or go to some graduate school in China. I didn't really want to go to take the graduate school entrance exam in China, so I thought I should go abroad. I mainly applied to schools in Hong Kong and Singapore. The master's programs in these two regions are shorter, lasting basically only one year. Meanwhile, they are closer to home. There will not be too much time difference and it will be more convenient to contact my family. At that time, I applied to the top 5 universities in Hong Kong and the top 2 in Singapore. In the first half of my senior year, I got offers from the Chinese University of Hong Kong (CUHK) and the Hong Kong University of Science and Technology, and then from the City University of Hong Kong. The University of Hong Kong was the only one that rejected me. (laughs) But at that time it was, I cannot remember clearly but you know, Hong Kong was in riots for a while. The students from CUHK were fighting for the independence of Hong Kong, and people from mainland China were too afraid to go there. Many other students who got offers from Hong Kong universities were also hesitating whether to go.

[00:03:22.11] Lily: 后来就,我想一想大概是什么时候。就是大四刚开学,大概是10月底的时候,因为我们这一批要毕业了,辅导员会在群里面发各种招聘信息、就业信息之类的。他有一天发了一个国家某某政委,某政委的一个什么宣讲会,大家就觉得特别神秘,不知道这个是干嘛的。后来了解了一下,其实是各级的[bi~~]来我们学校招应届,因为这个是涉及[bi~~]不能够面向社会招生,招的都是从学校里直接毕业的应届生直接招进去的。当时抱着一个好奇的心态去看了一下宣讲会,也投了一些简历出去,结果就过了浙江的[bi~~]的筛选。[bi~~]的考试,它是先进行一轮面试,这一轮面试我在学校是已经过了。它大概筛选出10个人左右参加一个岗位的考试,这个考试也就是公务员,跟公务员的省考试一体的,他们是考一张卷子。只能说这个岗位单独的,是不走社会报名的。它报名是单独的,但考试卷子是一体的。我当时跟家里人聊了之后,就说,反正也是一项就业机会嘛,就考一下吧,就开始准备公务员考试。后来准备了公务。大概11月的时候开始准备公务员考试。准备了之后才发现,原来公务员考试有很多种,有国考还有省考。那个时候其实之前完全没有了解过。它当年的考试的顺序,第一个是先考国考,国家公务员考试,第二个是江苏省的公务员考试,第三个才是浙江省的公务员考试。大概它日期上有一个先后差。这样子,当时反正我都复习了,因为大家考的都是一样的,内容是一样的,我就把国考和江苏的省考都考一下,抱着这种心态去报名了公务员考试。在考完江苏省的笔试之后,疫情爆发了。江苏省考试是19年12月份,大概考

完江苏省的考试之后，疫情爆发了。所以原本定在也是定在19年12月末的浙江省的考试就推迟了。当然，它后来一直推迟到20年的7月份。就是它推迟了这么长的时间。（笑）

And then, let me see when that was. At the beginning of my senior year, probably at the end of October, to help students find a job, the student instructor shared a lot of job descriptions in the WeChat group of our school. One day he posted information about a campus recruitment talk hosted by a government department. It didn't provide so much information and was very mysterious. Nobody knew what this was for. I asked for more details and was told it was all levels of [bi ~ ~] coming to our school to recruit fresh graduates because this government department is involved in [bi ~ ~], they were not able to recruit widely from the society. At that time, curiosity drove me to attend that recruitment talk and I did send some resumes out. And I passed the first round of selection of [bi ~ ~] in Zhejiang Province. The selection process of [bi~~] was like you had to have the first round of interviews at school and about 10 students would be selected. Then we would need to take the Civil Servant exam. More accurately, they were using the same papers as the Civil Servant exam of the particular province but recruiting separately, which meant we didn't need to compete with more examiners. After discussing it with my family, I thought it was an employment opportunity anyway, and I should have a try. So, in November, I started preparing for the Civil Servant Exam. When preparing for the exam, it was my first time knowing that there are different kinds of Civil Servant Exams, including one national exam and provincial exams hosted by different provinces. The exams take place at different times. The order of the exams that year was like the national exam came first, then the Jiangsu provincial exam, and Zhejiang provincial exam. There were gaps between the two exams. And I thought since the contents of the exams were the same and I had prepared for the Zhejiang exam, why not take the national and Jiangsu exams? With this idea in mind, I registered for the two exams. After taking the written exam in Jiangsu Province, the pandemic broke out. The Jiangsu provincial exam was on December 19, and the pandemic broke out shortly after. And the exam for Zhejiang province, which was originally scheduled at the end of December was postponed. In fact, it was postponed till July 2020. Such a long postpone! (laughs)

[00:06:06.26] Yiwen: 那个时候其实你已经有别的工作？

At that time, you have already found another job?

[00:06:10.14] Lily: 对，很奇怪。那一段时间。因为后来疫情，所以江苏省考和国考的面试也都推迟了。本来面试是定在2月份的。它成绩是照常出的。面试定在了2月份，但那个时候都知道疫情比较严重，基本上是举办不了的，到最后推迟了，我记得江苏的省考面试是定在了六月七号。我记得很清楚，因为它面试的前一天，6月6号，刚好是我本科毕业论文的线上答辩。6月6号我本科论文答辩完了之后，6月7号就去考面试了。因为面试的分数是当场出来的，不像笔试它需要批卷子，它的面试分数是考完了之后，考官就会当场扣分，你在考场外等一下，你就知道你的分数了。大概这个样子。所以考完面试，在跟同岗位的竞争者交流了一下之后，当场你能够知道结果。考完当天就知道应该是进了江苏省考，因为江苏应该是率先恢复面试的，好像是全国第一个。

Yes, it was a chaotic time. And because of the pandemic, the interviews for the Jiangsu and national exams were also postponed. The interview was originally scheduled in February. I received the results of the written exams on time. But for the interview in February, you know how serious the pandemic was in February and it was definitely impossible to hold interviews at that time. So, they postponed the interviews, and the Jiangsu one took place on June 7. I remember the date very clearly because the day before the interview, June 6, happened to be the day of the online defense of my undergraduate thesis. One day after my undergraduate thesis defense, I attended the Jiangsu interview. We were informed of the interview results instantly. Unlike the written exam, you need to wait for the papers to be graded, you can know the score right after the interview. So after the interview, after talking to my competitors, I was able to know the result that I passed the Jiangsu Provincial Exam and got the job I applied. And Jiangsu should be the first province to hold this interview.

[00:07:17.08] Lily: 紧接着是国考的面试，国考是在6月二十几号。那个时候我一开始是报名的，但是后来我放弃了。因为那个时候我们学校顶着压力把我们20级的，20届的毕业生叫回来参加毕业典礼，顶着疫情防控的压力，还是给我们办了毕业典礼。国考面试那天就刚好跟毕业典礼那天就撞了日期。我就打电话跟招考部门说就不去了。还蛮严格的，就让我录一个视频。什么手里拿着本人的身份证。然后说我自愿放弃什么考试。（笑）邮箱发过去。

Then, it was the interview for the national exam, which was held in late June. I initially planned to attend this interview, but finally gave up. At that time, our school called back the students from the class of 2020 to participate in the graduation ceremony under the pressure of pandemic prevention and control. The day of the interview for the national exam happened to clash with the date of the graduation ceremony. I called the recruiting department and said I wouldn't go. It was quite strict that they let me film a video, holding my ID card and saying I voluntarily give up the interview (laughs) email, and email the video to them.

[00:07:56.19] Lily: 也是在6月。你知道6月十几号的时候，我江苏省考已经通过了之后，我收到了南阳理工大学的offer。诶，这个事情当时真的6月份挤在一起了。我当时也很纠结到底要不要出去。6月份的时候他很奇怪，他6月十几号才给我发offer，然后要我立刻就办签证到学校去。好像当时是到了新加坡还是要隔离的，然后他9月份就要开学了。当时时间很紧，不能够，我也不能确定签证什么能不能办下来的，感觉非常的匆忙。当时也是咨询了一些身边的同学，老师还有家人们。基本上同学都是希望我，都觉得我应该继续去读书，家人都希望我留在[bi～～]工作这样。当然现在还是选择留在[bi～～]，参加了工作，也没有再去考浙江的考试。他7月份发过来的时候，我已经一切都结束了。（笑）

And it was also in June. I received an offer from Nanyang University of Technology after I had passed the Jiangsu Provincial Exam on the 10th of June. Everything really happened at almost the same time. I was very torn about whether to go or not. And it was strange that they sent me an offer in mid-June but asked me to apply for a visa as soon as possible. I remember at that time, a quarantine was still needed when you entered Singapore. The school would begin in September and that was such a hurry. I was not so sure whether I could get the visa and enroll in time. So I consulted some of my classmates, teachers, and family members. Basically, my classmates all suggested I go to Singapore, and my family wanted me to stay [bi~~] and work. Finally, I chose to stay in [bi~~] and began working. And of course, I did not take the Zhejiang exam. When they sent me the notification in July, everything had settled down. (laughs)

[00:09:02.11] Yiwen: 你当时自己会有一个偏向性吗？虽然你咨询了很多人，但是你看同学希望你出去读书，但是家人希望你留在家乡工作。

Did you have a preference yourself? You see, you consulted so many people and your classmates thought going abroad would be better while your family preferred you to go back to your hometown and work.

[00:09:12.02] Lily: 我当时肯定还是偏向于去读书的。这个事情怎么说？一方面当时的环境，现在的防疫政策就不多说了，当时的疫情环境，国内主流的风声还是，国内的疫情防控做得比较好，国外的环境比较的危险。包括当时国际上，据我了解，可能一些反华的情绪还是比较严重的。对，包括新加坡也有一些，这个样子。当然能读书还是读书好，我觉得还是读书比较好。（smile bitterly)

I definitely preferred to go to school. But how to say. On one hand, the atmosphere at that time, I would not comment on the pandemic prevention and control policy now, but at that time, the mainstream view was the policy in China was better and all the places outside of China would be dangerous. Meanwhile, as I knew, in many countries, including Singapore, the anti-Chinese sentiment was relatively strong. But in any case, it's always better to go to school if you can, I think.

[00:09:52.27] Yiwen: 那你现在喜欢你的工作吗？

So, do you like your job now?

[00:09:54.09] Lily: 嗯…工作？工作这个事情，工作，你没有办法说喜欢或者讨厌或者什么，它其实你生活当中要完成的一个部分，他给你钱，你做事，我觉得这样的一个关系，对他也没有什么期待。说实话。

Emm…my job? You cannot say you like or do not like your job. It's just an essential part of your life. They pay for you, and you work for them. I think this is my relationship with my job. I really have no exception on it, to be honest.

[00:10:19.16] Yiwen: 你现在再回看你 2020 年的时候当时遇到的状态，你会选择去读书还是留下来工作？

So if you look back on your life in 2020, would you choose to go to Singapore or stay at home working?

[00:10:28.06] Lily: 这个问题其实，其实确实想过很多次。但是因为我可能从小就是听家长的话比较多的那种类型，我想了想，如果同样的事情摆在面前，我可能还是会选择工作，因为公务员他确实是一个，就是你没有什么盼头，但却特别稳定稳定的那种工作类型。嗯，而且现在考公，国内考公的相当于热潮吧，反正疫情以来越来越热，报考的人也越来越多。如果我真的当年去读一年硕士回来，当然，我当时的规划里也没有读完硕士回来考公务员，可能希更希望留在大城市，然后进入大厂这样的一个路线，因为我大部分同学也都是这个样子的。但是想了想，如果我读完一年硕士回来再考公务员，也不能确定能不能够考上了。

This question, in fact, I did think about it many times. But because I might be the type of person growing up obedient to my parents, if I could have a second chance, I may still make the same choice. Because civil servant is the kind of job that you have nothing to look forward to, but very stable. Well, now, especially after the pandemic, it's becoming more and more popular among young people, and more and more people are taking the civil servant exams every year. If I really went to study for a master's degree and came back one year later, of course, I never thought about pursuing a master's degree and coming back to work as a civil servant, my initial plan was to stay in a big city and work in a big company, which is the routine of most of my classmates. But if I really take that exam after getting my master's degree, I'm not sure if I can get the same job.

[00:11:40.25] VoiceOver: 在采访中，Lily 还与我探讨了工作一段时间后再重返校园的话题。

In the interview, Lily also discussed the topic of returning to campus after working for some time.

[00:11:46.24] Yiwen: 你会考虑再比如说重新申请，比如新加坡或者新香港的研究生，再考虑辞职出去读书吗？

Will you consider re-applying to some master's programs in Singapore or Hong Kong, and quit your job to go back to school?

[00:11:55.19] Lily: 我应该不会考虑这个选项。因为工作之后，家里也是帮我买了车和房子。我现在的工资肯定是要还贷的。如果我辞职了再出去读书，一个是，就

是它会断供，你的贷款会断供。一个是我工作以来也一直在还车贷，基本上每个月的工资还完车贷，也剩的不是很多，所以也并没有很多的存款去支撑我去读书了。

I may not. Because after I got this job, my parents bought a new car and a new apartment for me. Now, I need to use part of my salary to pay off the loan. If I quit the job to go back to school, on one hand, I would face a loan interruption. And on the other hand, I'm paying off the loan of my car on my own, and my salary is not much left after paying off the loan. So, I also don't have enough savings to pay for the tuition.

[00:12:29.20] Yiwen: 那你之后会考虑比如说再去读一个在职的这样子的研究生吗？或者是这一类。

So, would you consider applying for a part-time graduate program in China?

[00:12:37.23] Lily: 对，我其实正在准备。因为我当时是了解了一下国内的在职研究生，它是需要本科毕业3年之后才可以考的。所以我工作的前两年没有准备，现在我应该算毕业的第二年。但是如果我考上的话，去读的时候，就刚好本科毕业满三年了。大概是这样的。所以我其实近期也在准备考在职的硕士，就准备考研吧。

（Laugh）

Yes. Actually, I'm preparing for it. As I know, if you want to enter a part-time graduate program in China, you have to graduate from college for at least 3 years. So I didn't apply for it in the first two years of working. Now, it's still the second year after my graduating. But if I can get an offer, I will have already graduated for three years. And this is the situation I'm facing. So, I'm preparing for the graduate school entrance exam in China recently. (Laugh.)

[00:13:13.29] Yiwen: 那你觉得工作一段时间，再去进行一个所谓的学历的提升，和这种无缝衔接的，在本科毕业之后直接去读研究生，你个人感觉会不太一样吗？So, how do you think about the difference between pursuing a master's degree several years after graduating from college and attending a master's program right after graduation?

[00:13:29.29] Lily: 很不一样，我觉得。因为我觉得你本科毕业之后读的硕士，它是一个比较纯粹的上学的过程，你可以还有很多不同的方向可以选择。比如说，我读硕士的时候有什么感兴趣的，我可以再去进行学术研究，或者我不再研究这个，但我可以去拓展我以后进行一个什么方向。就是你人生可能会有更多方向的选择。但工作之后再去读硕士，大家基本上单纯地为了一个文凭这个样子，没有更多的考虑了。它可以选择的专业也很少，就公共管理，工商管理这些。

I think it would be quite different. For me, attending a master's program right after graduation can be a relatively pure process of studying. And you can have much more choices, like you may keep doing some academic research if you find something interesting during this period. Or even if you don't want to do research, you can start your career related to it. It means you can have more possibilities in your life. But pursuing a master's degree usually only means a promotion in your educational background, and what most of your classmates want is only the diploma. Furthermore, the programs you can apply for are limited, mostly Public Administration (MPA) or Business Administration (MBA).

[00:14:16.15] (Music)

Reflective essay

Dealing with different interviewees

For this project, I have conducted 8 interviews in total. And recently, I'm working on another oral history project on the life story of Chinese students who entered top universities from rural areas after the resumption of college entrance examinations. For that project, I conducted 16 interviews with 6 narrators.

When conducting these interviews, I found the personality of the narrators can greatly influence the effectiveness of the interview. As interviewers, we need to adopt different interview strategies and respond differently according to the characteristics of each interviewee.

For narrators like Keke and Zoey, ask them an open-ended question, and they would give you a speech, organized and informative. As an interviewer, somehow your work would be very easy. The only thing I needed to do was to give out questions following my interview guide and occasionally raise some follow-up questions. Even the editing process was so smooth that I could easily get relatively complete clips, without the need to cut out too many short pieces to make the podcast sound clean.

For narrators like Evan, they prefer to give very short answers to even very open-ended questions. As the interviewer, I would keep asking follow-up questions or reminding them of giving me more details. These follow-up questions are acceptable for archived oral history, but for a podcast, the audience may feel it not so coherent. Some more efforts are needed for editing.

Then, narrators like 71 can be another type. They need more time for thinking and long silences often occur during the interview with them because before giving any narrative they will self-evaluate on whether the story is worthy to be the main content of a podcast. They would even filter out some experiences for they were not interesting enough or not unique enough and tell you they have nothing special to share about this question. When interviewing 71, I took the strategy of sharing some of my own experiences to inspire her. This worked for her because we have similar backgrounds, so I could find stories to share with her. However, if the interviewee is a complete stranger and I have no life experience related to the topic, what should I do to open my interviewee? This is a question I am still thinking about and needs more practice to find an answer.

There is another kind of interviewee that does not exist in any of the interviews I did for this project, but I met them when conducting interviews for the other project I mentioned above. She is a college teacher and scholar who did quite a lot of research on students from rural China. She knows the field much better than I do. Of course, she has her own analytical framework and narrative system. After I asked the first question, she began her "speech" on her life story. I tried to interrupt her to regain control of the interview, only to find that her narrative contained everything I wanted to get and was even more detailed. For a moment, I felt like I was just an assistant operating the recorder for her. As an oral historian, I need to "open up narrative spaces" for my narrators and give them the opportunity to "volunteer stories of their own" (Portelli, "Living Voices: The Oral History Interview as Dialogue and Experience" 243), but where are the boundaries? Would such an interview be considered an oral history if the interviewer plays almost exclusively a recording role through the entire interview?

Some of my audience also found this problem. One of them, who is also my friend, JJ thought some of the interviews were lack of interactivity and control of the pacing. This didn't mean the content of the podcast was uninteresting, but it left him feeling like it was the interviewee taking the wheel and that I didn't succeed in playing the role of a host as well as I should have. He pointed out that the most out-of-control episode was the interview with Keke. However, before getting the comments from him, among all the interviews I did for this project, my favorite part was Keke's narrative about her life during the lockdown in Wuhan. It is actually not so relevant to the subject of my project, but for the final version to be released in the podcast, I still kept part of it due to my preference.

In fact, when I was designing my interview guidance, I didn't list any questions about the situation in Wuhan in early 2020, nor the life of my narrator during the lockdown. However, when conducting the interview with Keke, considering her identity as a Wuhaner, as a greeting and an introduction leading to the main part of the interview, I asked the question, "Do you still remember what the overall situation was like in Wuhan at that time?" Keke is a very talkative narrator, and she delivered a very detailed description of how the pandemic developed in Wuhan and how her mood changed at the time. Her narrative was so vivid and engaging that I totally forgot my interview guidance and began to ask follow-up questions on this topic, which should not be the keystone of my interview. Afterward, when I listened back to this interview, I immediately realized the problem--a large part of our interview had deviated from the original plan.

However, I just loved this unplanned part of the interview so much. When editing the podcast, I gave myself 101 excuses to keep this part, like it's interesting and meaningful, and no one would refuse to listen to a narrative from someone who experienced the lockdown in Wuhan entirely. As you can see, although I have unwillingly deleted the part about food, I kept most of Keke's stories about Wuhan during the lockdown in the podcast. In addition, I'm still thinking about adding that part as a special episode.

Interestingly, it is not the first time I lost control in an interview. When conducting an interview for the Missing Them project[8], our conversation also had a sudden shift to his parents' early experiences as immigrants after the interviewee's mentioning of his father's identity as a paper son, yet the interview was intended to be focused on his brother's life history.

I tried to find some solutions to this problem and I found a blog on transom.org on losing control in an interview. The author Erica Heilman suggested:

> You might not get to anything really great if you're scared to guide the conversation. Yes, you want your interviewee to feel comfortable. But if he doesn't stop talking about his blue heeler you're going to run out of time and you don't want the blue heeler tape. Interrupt with enthusiasm and love. 'I really want

---

[8] It is an online obituary project designed to memorize New Yorkers who lost their lives because of Covid-19. By interviewing their loved ones and friends, we get to know their life stories and then write obituaries for them.

> to hear more about . . .' 'Can we talk about . . .?' 'I'm going to take a hard right here and ask you about . . .' You can guide the conversation. People are less fragile than you think. (Heilman)

Although it seems to make some sense, I don't think it can be achieved in practice. The situations I met do have some similarities in that I felt the topic my narrators were talking about was attractive and I was eager to know more about it. Under the circumstances, how could I think of interrupting my interviewees?

I'm not sure whether conducting more interviews would be effective in solving this problem. But perhaps, at this stage, the only thing I can do is to comfort myself with another quote from this author:

> It is difficult to have a good interview if you are following a list of questions. You can have the list. Just don't take it out of your bag. Toward the end, if you want to have a look at the list, have a look at the list. (Heilman)

Relationship with my narrators

When designing this project, I intentionally chose to do oral history with my high school or college friends for the following reasons:

1. The narrators and I have known each other for so many years, so we can save time to get familiar with each other, enter the conversation more easily, and create a more relaxed atmosphere. The narrators may be more willing to tell their true thoughts.
2. The narrators and I have similar backgrounds and experiences, so it may be easier to resonate with each other in the conversation. At the same time, we may see things from different perspectives, and such conversations may also give us some inspiration.
3. Through some pre-surveys, I found that these friends of mine, despite having faced very similar situations, made very different choices. In my friend circle, diversity was formed that I believe can make my project representative of a certain group of people. Before sending out the invitation letters, I did make a list of potential interviewees. My primary consideration in selecting interviewees is whether there are points to be explored in them. (Sounds like a journalist, right?)

And during the preparation process, my ideal atmosphere for my podcast should be very similar to the episode "Goodbye Xiaolu 再见小鹿" from *Stochastic Volatility* (Fu et al.), which is one of my favorite Chinese podcasts. It is relaxing, warming, and engaging. I attribute their success in creating this atmosphere to the fact that the hosts and the guest are familiar with each other. But one thing I overlooked is that, aside from the fact that all three hosts are veteran media people, the guest Xiaolu is also a very well-known stand-up comedian. They're all very familiar with and good at public speaking, and that's probably where the relaxing atmosphere of this podcast comes from. My interviewees and I, on the contrary, clearly do not have such qualifications.

Of course, our weakness at public speaking may not be the only reason for the less-than-expected atmosphere. I found that even if all the interviewees are close friends with me, the way how the interview was conducted could also influence the performance of the interview. I did my interviews with a combination of remote and in-person formats. This mostly depended on the distance between the interviewee and me. Under this circumstance, I did feel the superiority of the face-to-face interview.

Although the HD cameras and increasingly advanced online conferencing software allow us to also see the interviewees' facial expressions and record the interviews clearly, when sitting in the same room, "the interviewer is exposed not only to the narrative but also to the private space of the interviewee and can read his or her body language" (Livne and Bejarano 187). Only in contrast to remote interviewing did I feel the importance of body language in oral history. Face-to-face communication is indeed more helpful in understanding my narrators and creating the engaging atmosphere I wanted.

Furthermore, the similarity of my experiences and backgrounds with my interviewees did make it easier for me to resonate with them that I could also share my own stories as a supplement, but it also led to some homogenization of content in each podcast episode. Although I specifically selected interviewees who made different choices in 2020 at the beginning, this diversity did not seem sufficient. As my outside advisor, Dian Zi once pointed out, my interviewees all graduated from top universities in

China and their stories and experience may not be relevant enough to the general public. I totally understand Dian's point, but I don't think it will be a problem. I think this homogenization otherwise makes us more of a whole. In other words, it makes the content of this podcast more focused and representative.

So, at least for me, starting this podcast by sharing the experiences and thoughts of a small group of people was the right choice overall. But if I continue to work on this project in the future, I may consider expanding the source of interviewees to some strangers with more diverse backgrounds.

Self-censorship in China

I don't want to talk too much about the official censorship in China here, though after I submit each episode on the podcast platform, I need to wait for it to be previewed by their staff in case any content touches the political red line. This is not consistent with Siobhán McHugh's claim that podcasts can bypass China's censorship by avoiding AI facial recognition and 'offensive' image detection. (McHugh, 223-224) And naturally, as people grow up in China, my friends are all aware of how to avoid this kind of trouble. They have shown a high level of self-censorship in their interviews, for example by actively avoiding commenting on any China's current policy.

Their self-censorship is also reflected in their deep understanding of the Chinese Internet environment. It is interesting that in China, those who have relatively better educational backgrounds would be seen as elite, and the general public would be curious about their life. However, this curiosity is not always in a good way. I sometimes call myself a Chinese Internet watcher. And from my observations, this group will be judged more often for what they say on the Internet. When what they say meets most netizens' imagination and expectations, or is consistent with their perceptions, they would receive praises like, "No wonder you're a graduate of a top university!" However, once their words are less satisfying, their educational background, especially the experience of studying abroad, can instead become the original sin.

Under the self-censorship for these two situations, when conducting the interviews, I can feel the cautiousness of my interviewees that they would immediately remind me to "cut this out" when they unconsciously said something they thought might be sensitive. For example, both Zoey and Lily had asked me to remove some of their comments about China's quarantine policy. After finishing the editing, I would also send the audio to my narrators as requested and discuss with them if there is still anything that needs to be cut because it might be controversial. Self-censorship seems to be a basic skill for everyone who grew up in China.

Oral history and podcast

After deciding to produce an oral history podcast as my final project, I tried to find a suitable example to use as a reference. And I did find one, *America Works*, which was first launched in 2020 by the American Folklife Center (AFC). The whole series is available on Apple Podcasts, Stitcher, and on the website of the Library of Congress at https://www.loc.gov/podcasts/america-works/. (*America Works*) Since the first episode was released in 2020, the series has come to the third season and updated to the 25th episode. Each episode of this podcast series averages 10 minutes in length and "is based on an interview from the AFC's ongoing *Occupational Folklife Project*." (Tucker)

It is worth noticing that the host of this podcast series is Nancy Groce, the senior folklife specialist at AFC. And her other role is the project director of the oral history project *Occupational Folklife Project.* This oral history project was launched 10 years earlier than the podcast series and is still ongoing. To date, this collection has included more than 1300 oral history interviews with workers from all walks of life across the United State. Each interview lasts for 50-60 minutes and "features workers discussing their current jobs and formative work experiences, reflecting on their training, on-the-job challenges and rewards, aspirations, and occupational communities." All the interviews were archived in LOC and were divided into different collections based on their topics. Among them, 26 collections with 622 interviews are currently online, and the audiences can access those interviews at https://www.loc.gov/collections/occupational-folklife-project/. ("Occupational Folklife Project")

From this, it is easy to see that the strategy Nancy has adopted is to select some from all the oral history interviews she has archived and edit them into a podcast. Though the length of each episode is a little more than 10 minutes, excluding the introduction parts, the actual body of the podcast is quite short, especially compared with the one-hour raw materials. The podcast team sees this podcast series as "a better, smarter, more flexible platform that allows us to easily retrieve and share collection data."(Groce and Lyons)

When I was working on my podcast, I borrowed the length from Nancy. Each of my interviews is about two hours long, but I don't think most audience would have the patience for such a long podcast. My initial plan was to keep the length of each episode around 15 minutes, which is the length I picked after conducting a small survey among my Chinese friends. We wanted this podcast series to be one that allows people to use their pocket time to get some small pieces of information. One thing that differs from *America works* is that based on the discussions with my interviewees, I finally decided not to archive the full interviews. The podcast ends where it is and the listeners cannot find a more complete interview in any other place. This required me and my interviewees to be able to pick the most critical elements of the interview in the podcast. However, the 15-minute plan was broken in the second episode, and I ended up keeping each episode under 25 minutes. Although this length is still not very difficult for most audience to finish an entire episode in one time, the lack of consistency in the time may make the audience confused (Rios). This is something I need to keep in mind if I'm going to produce a new podcast series in the future.

I did find some similarities between podcasts and oral history. In Richard Baker's case of producing the podcast *The Age*, I learned that narrators would have more self-consciousness when listening to their own voices than reading printed words. In order to prevent interviewees from questioning the content after the podcast has been released, he chose to give the transcript to the interviewees for preview in advance, which he would not have done for a print article. (McHugh, 178) Although one is open to the public and the other is usually only accessible to a small number of researchers, the protection of interviewees and the avoidance of subsequent risks make podcasts and oral histories overlap to some extent.

One difference between oral histories and podcast audio is that podcasts need to provide the most comfortable listening experience we can. (Rios) In oral histories, it is necessary to preserve the interviewees' thought processes, pauses, and constant correction of their own words. However, podcasts are expected to be more clear-cut for the more general audience would not have so much patience figuring out and extracting useful information from a piece of audio full of interjections and corrections of previous context. Since what I am producing, anyway, is an oral history podcast, I hope to retain some of the qualities of oral history in the final version without compromising the audience's understanding. In the first two episodes, I retained all the conventions of oral history, not only in audio, but also in my transcriptions and the translated version, but I overestimated how receptive most audience would be to so much "emm" in the transcriptions as non-oral historians. So, after repeated rethinking, I continued to keep the "emm" and pauses that indicate thought as much as possible in the audio of the last three episodes, but weakened them in the transcriptions. I think this is a reasonable compromise and balance.

www.ingramcontent.com/pod-product-compliance
Lightning Source LLC
LaVergne TN
LVHW020443070526
838199LV00063B/4838